"Sometimes the very best contribution that Christians can make to contemporary public policy disputes is to refuse to engage them according to the terms available in the culture, but instead to return to the riches of our own tradition. That is what Willard Swartley has done so splendidly in this new book. Grounded in personal as well as ecclesial experiences, Swartley engages Scripture, Christian history and mission, and the vexatious problems associated with health care in our own context to offer sober, mature and constructive treatment of a critical issue that has been obscured by being caught up in the partisan vortex. Highly recommended as a work at the intersection of Scripture, mission and Christian ethics."

David P. Gushee, Distinguished University Professor of Christian Ethics, director, Center for Theology and Public Life, Mercer University

"Finally a resource to reflect biblically, theologically and morally about the pressing need for health care reform in the United States. *Health, Healing and the Church's Mission* offers us hopeful and grace-filled ways to think about the extension of Jesus' healing ministry through the practices and commitments of the church. Professor Swartley reminds us these conversations cannot be abstract and aloof. People's lives are at stake."

Wyndy Corbin Reuschling, professor of ethics and theology, Ashland Theological Seminary

"Willard Swartley has done the Christian community a huge service by writing a comprehensive, thoughtful and lucid discussion on our biblical and moral responsibility to promote healing and to advocate for a just health care system. His argument goes beyond the usual economic, political and medical arenas by focusing on Christian healing, community and mission."

Mary McDonough, author of *Can a Health Market Be Moral? A Catholic Vision*

"With an eloquent, rational approach, Willard Swartley critiques the current health care industry and persuasively offers a substantive alternative insight into health and healing by incorporating insights from Scripture, varied cultures, historic and religious practices, and contemporary trends. Swartley advances and amplifies the concept of shalom that embodies holistic health and reflects the biblical view of health. This vital and important volume will be valued by health care workers who aspire to experience how Christian faith can meaningfully transform their understanding and practice. I look forward to using this resource as a textbook for students in our biomedicine program."

Roman J. Miller, Eastern Mennonite University

"Health, Healing and the Church's Mission is a unique and refreshing contribution to the discussion of health, healing and the provision of health care. Swartley offers a comprehensive biblical perspective and fosters a welcome discussion of the moral dilemmas we all feel. An important read for any person of faith seeking a biblical grounding on these issues."
Christine Sine, author and executive director of Mustard Seed Associates

"Dr. Swartley clearly articulates the profound moral challenges facing the Christian church in response to many of the dilemmas of health care services in America. He does so through the lenses of a thoughtful treatment of biblical and theological perspectives and the rich history of Judeo-Christian engagement in health ministries of many forms. He highlights various alternative models of health services that may offer hope. This book is must reading for religious and institutional health care leaders who are willing to examine and are open to re-claiming the essence of God's reconciling and healing work in this world."
Rick Stiffney, president/CEO, Mennonite Health Services Alliance

"Swartley's holistic approach to the issue of health gives fresh perspectives on both healing in the Christian tradition and current issues of health care reform. Readers who are looking for ways to integrate contemporary questions about health care with a biblical and theological perspective that moves from text to tradition will find many valuable resources in Swartley's work."
Mary Veeneman, North Park University

To Carl Yoder
Blessings to you in your
CHH & medical ministry.
3 John 2

WILLARD M. SWARTLEY

Willard Swartley
Oct. 2, 2012

Health, Healing
and the
Church's
Mission

Biblical Perspectives
and Moral Priorities

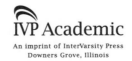

IVP Academic
An imprint of InterVarsity Press
Downers Grove, Illinois

InterVarsity Press
P.O. Box 1400, Downers Grove, IL 60515-1426
World Wide Web: www.ivpress.com
E-mail: email@ivpress.com

InterVarsity Press® is the book-publishing division of InterVarsity Christian Fellowship/USA®, a movement of students and faculty active on campus at hundreds of universities, colleges and schools of nursing in the United States of America, and a member movement of the International Fellowship of Evangelical Students. For information about local and regional activities, write Public Relations Dept., InterVarsity Christian Fellowship/USA, 6400 Schroeder Rd., P.O. Box 7895, Madison, WI 53707-7895, or visit the IVCF website at <www.intervarsity.org>.

Scripture quotations, unless otherwise noted, are from the New Revised Standard Version of the Bible, *copyright 1989 by the Division of Christian Education of the National Council of the Churches of Christ in the USA. Used by permission. All rights reserved.*

While all stories in this book are true, some names and identifying information in this book have been changed to protect the privacy of the individuals involved.

The words to "I Worship You, O Lord" are by James E. Seddon, © *The Jubilate Group (Admin. Hope Publishing Company, Carol Stream, IL 60188). All rights reserved. Used by permission. The addition to this hymn by Calvin Seerveld is used courtesy of Calvin Seerveld <www.seerveld.com/tuppence.html>.*

Quotes from Jean Vanier originally appeared in The Church and the Disabled, *published by Templegate Publishers in 1983 and used courtesy of Griff Hogan.*

"Midnight Prayer" and "Hold Me, Lord" from Henry Swartley's Living on the Fault-Line *are used courtesy of Willard Swartley.*

The words to "O Christ, the Healer," are by Fred Pratt Green, © *1969 Hope Publishing Company, Carol Stream, IL 60188. All rights reserved. Used by permission.*

"Nine Maxims on Suffering" is used courtesy of Reverend Cornel G. Rempel, director of pastoral services and CPE supervisor, Philhaven, Mt. Gretna, Pennsylvania.

Figure 7.2 by George Panikulam is from Koinōnia in the New Testament: A Dynamic Expression of Christian Life *in the series Analecta Biblica 85, and it is used courtesy of Biblical Institute Press, Rome.*

Portion of "Hard Rock into Springs of Water: Working in Hope," is used courtesy of Tim Leaman, M.D., from Mennonite Health Journal *11, no. 3 (July-Sept. 2009): 24-25.*

Cover design: Cindy Kiple
Interior design: Beth Hagenberg
Images: © *Ragnarocks/iStockphoto*

ISBN 978-0-8308-3974-2

Printed in the United States of America ∞

Library of Congress Cataloging-in-Publication Data

Swartley, Willard M., 1936-
  Health, healing and the church's mission: Biblical perspectives and moral priorities / Willard M. Swartley.
    p. cm.
  Includes bibliographical references and index.
  ISBN 978-0-8308-3974-2 (pbk. : alk. paper)
  1. Healing—Religious aspects—Christianity. 2. Healing—Biblical teaching. 3. Health—Religious aspects—Christianity. 4. Medical care—Religious aspects—Christianity. I. Title.
  BT732.S925 2012
  261.8'321—dc23

                                                                    2012018670

P	20	19	18	17	16	15	14	13	12	11	10	9	8	7	6	5	4	3	2	1
Y	29	28	27	26	25	24	23	22	21	20	19	18	17	16	15	14	13	12			

In memory, to my parents and siblings:

William Henry and Ida Swartley

Kenneth, Henry, Clifford, Emerson, Marian

And to those who remain: Dorothy and John

All who nurtured me with love

Contents

Tables and Diagrams

Preface

Writing on health and healing is a daunting task. Amid the dominant health care debates today, a book on health and healing in Scripture and the Christian church's commitment to health care over the centuries may relegate this study to narrative archaeology. Nonetheless, if the church is to be faithful to its source, Jesus Christ, we cannot camouflage Jesus' dual mission of healing and proclaiming the kingdom of God. The topic faces us with the pressing existential realities of sickness, suffering and dying as well. What does love for one another, prayer for ourselves and others when ill, and caring for the sick mean for us in today's world? This book addresses these topics.

With necessary limits for such topical scope, this book focuses on the church's mission in health and healing. It calls the Christian church to own its biblical, historical and theological heritage and its mission in healing and health care. It challenges the current dominant assumption that health care is an economic, political or medical issue only. It regards U.S. health care a moral priority. May it stimulate discussion!

I owe special gratitude to readers and helpers in bringing this work to fruition. I thank Philip Yoder, minister and seminary graduate with interest in healing, health care and mission. Philip read chapters in their initial stages and wisely suggested I include a historical overview of the church's healing ministry (thus chap. 8). Similarly, Amy Jo Jones, a hospice chaplain in Oregon and former student at the Anabaptist Mennonite Biblical Seminary (hereafter AMBS), read most of the manuscript, with suggestions for improvement. Her out-of-the-blue e-mail to me one day began the conversation, resulting in her wise counsel. I am indebted to Jenn

Burkett, director of Total Value Management at Elkhart General Hospital, for her suggestions regarding the present health care challenge and helping me construct categories of expression at home among health care professionals (chap. 10). I am grateful for the constructive critique of parts of this book by six medical doctors in my church, Belmont Mennonite: Eben Kio (oncology), Sally Krabill (family practice), Josh Mathew (psychiatry), Ben Smucker (orthopaedic surgery), Jon Shenk (emergency medicine) and Jon Schrock (pain management). As chapter twelve shows, I am indebted to Dr. James Nelson Gingerich and Dr. Tim Leaman. My neighbor and professor emeritus at Fuller Theological Seminary, Wilbert Shenk, helped me with aspects of mission history, especially the Mennonite and Brethren in Christ story (appendix 1). My nephew, Dr. Herbert Myers, retired psychiatrist, made many helpful suggestions. John A. Lapp kindly read the manuscript and helped with accuracy on certain points, as well as several infelicities, and to Willard Roth for his counsel on several editorial matters. I am grateful to Rick Stiffney (CEO for Mennonite Health Services Alliance) for helping me understand how this alliance of health-related institutions contributes to numerous dimensions of health care. Thanks also to Rick for connecting me to numerous denominational leaders in health/health care ministries, who commend this book. Other professionals (theological and medical) contributed insights as well, for which I am grateful.

I express special thanks to Gary Deddo, senior editor at InterVarsity Press, for his guidance from beginning to end in making a manuscript into this book. With patience, good will and blessing, he accepted "additions" between the usual back-and-forth transmissions of the manuscript. I am grateful for the outside reader whose perceptive comments strengthen the book significantly. My thanks also go to Drew Blankman for his editorial work and to Caitie Johnston who at an early stage managed preparation for sales and marketing of the book. Thanks to those who did the typesetting and proofreading of the page proofs. I am grateful also for the publishers and persons who granted permission to utilize key quotations or diagrams that enrich this book.

Above all, thanks be to God/Jesus Christ/Holy Spirit, from whom all healing flows!

Introduction

On an ordinary early fall morning I read a most fascinating story in our local newspaper. It reported the mysterious, miraculous healing of a quadriplegic person in a nearby town, Bristol, Indiana. Laura Nauman, who suffered for five years from a degenerative disorder of the nervous system, diagnosed in 1991 as "spinal muscular atrophy," woke up September 2, 1995, able to walk. The *(Elkhart) Truth* (October 1, 1995) reported Laura's unprecedented healing, quoting words of amazement from her doctor, Bristol physician Alan H. Bierlein, and First Baptist Church pastor John Blodgett. Both went to her home on Saturday, the morning of the new Laura, and during the next nine hours watched her walk, drive a four-wheeler and ride in a convertible. A related *Truth* article narrated her church's response when on the next Sunday morning her pastor mentioned her name, and one person thought, *Oh, she must have died.* But instead Laura got up out of her familiar wheel chair and bounded across the platform to the congregation's amazement, clapping and praising the Lord. The healing is inexplicable. Whether Laura or church people were praying for miraculous healing was not indicated. The miracle was a gift of God's lavish love and generous grace. In several other recent cases where medical specialists expected a person to die within a week or two, the person lives! One story cited in chapter eight, note one, also illustrates the miraculous.

But what about the majority who live with debilitating illnesses and are not cured, even though many prayers ascend to our Creator and Savior God for healing? This perplexity riddles this book. My denominational churchwide mission statement is:

God calls us as followers of Jesus Christ and,
by the power of the Holy Spirit,
to grow to be communities of grace, joy, and peace,
so that God's healing and hope
flow through us to the world. [1]

God's "healing and hope"—what does that mean? My own near-death heart illness is not fully healed, though I live, love, care, write and pray. The apostle Paul calls us to hope that goes beyond our present infirmities (Rom 5:1-3; Phil 3:10-12; 1 Cor 15). Can we affirm this mission statement without the hope that our bodies will be healed through resurrection, with its glimpses in history and fulfillment at the end of time? I think not— *except* when God surprises us to alert us to the kingdom in its fullness dawning even now in the "not yet" time. These texts remind us that resurrection hope points us beyond our own best efforts, toward the "heavenly call of God in Christ Jesus." In the Ash Wednesday ritual we are reminded of our mortality: "dust we are, and to dust we shall return." This is a necessary stance from which to begin. With resurrection hope, however, our thinking and acting in healing and health care ends not with Ash Wednesday but with Easter's hope and healing.

Why do I write a book on health, healing and the church's mission in the context of the present health care debates? These topics pose issues that baffle the best of minds and intimidate the heart's good will. My training is not in professional health care but in biblical studies, with a longstanding interest in healing, especially emotional and spiritual (including deliverance ministries in which I have witnessed "miracles" also). My contribution thus focuses on some hard questions raised by Scripture and how we understand healing from a biblical point of view. I affirm too the significant contribution of health care professionals to health and healing. Without those, this book would not be.

While one goal of the book is to help us respond with moral passion to the current health care challenges in the United States and maximize healing and shalom in our lives, its main purpose is to reclaim the relationship between the triune God and our healing and health care efforts. This requires explicating the biblical (Old and New Testaments) understandings of health

---

[1]Adopted by the Mennonite Church in its 1995 Assembly.

and healing, and assessing their ethical perspectives on healing and health care. The Christian church has been involved in health care since the church's inception. Given this tradition, we are called to reaffirm and encourage the church's present mission and ministry in healing and health care. A corollary purpose is to highlight the relation between God as healer—also Jesus as healer and the Spirit as healer—and the work of health care professionals, the many people in our churches who work in health care.

In many church congregations the Sunday morning worship service includes time for sharing. Members often request prayer for someone ill or facing a medical intervention. Why do we share these things in church? Only if we believe that the church body and its beliefs are integrally related to our health and well being does it make sense to do so. Gayle Gerber Koontz says in her editorial to essays on *Suffering*, "If this is not a place where tears are understood, then where can I go to cry?"[2] Some congregations, like my own, have designated Sundays when we have prayers for healing, when people come forward to request prayer for a given situation, and the pastor or elder prays for that person's need, while the congregation may stand, sing and pray.

Perhaps an even deeper reason why it makes sense for a congregation to include requests for healing in its sharing time is because in baptism we pledge to *care* for one another. *Praying* and *caring* are important practices enabling healing. Some church congregations include health care related activities: blood pressure clinics, nutrition seminars, Weight Watchers club, twelve-step programs and even free immunizations, with doctors and nurses on hand.

My Journey Toward This Book

As far back as the late 1970s when I was working on my book *Slavery, Sabbath, War, and Women*, I was thinking about healing, among other topics that might be treated to show that the Bible's voice on healing is not monovocal. Because Scripture at places says if we pray for healing when sick—or whatever we pray for—we should receive what we ask for. Yet at the same time the Bible is clear that humans suffer illness and die. Humans are mortal and bear the scars of fallen humanity and flawed creation.

---

[2]Gayle Gerber Koontz, editorial in *Suffering*; *Vision: A Journal for Church and Theology* 8, no. 2 (2007): 3.

Further, my longstanding interest in Scripture and healing has been complemented by an equally longstanding concern for the biblical teaching on and the church's practice of financially helping one another in times of sickness and other types of need. I addressed this topic in *Communities of Compassion* and speak to this issue in chapter seven of this book.[3] This combined agenda is the cradle of this contribution, as well as my journey toward healing from nearly dying from heart illness.

My heart attack in 1999 occurred when I was on a family retreat in the mountains of West Virginia. I did not recognize it as a heart attack because I did not associate severe indigestion with heart attack. That evening I was unusually tired and slept for three hours. Then I woke up and began throwing up (I thought my symptoms indicated food poisoning). Not until we began the drive to the hospital in Elkins did I feel any chest or arm pain. I was diagnosed with a massive heart attack. I was then flown by helicopter to the University of West Virginia hospital, where the cardiologist implanted a stent in my left artery descending. However, five hours had elapsed. Consequently I live with a 50 percent or more heart muscle loss that curbs my lifestyle.

The current health crisis and later interventions during the last twelve years inform and temper my perspectives. My experience illustrates the need for better self-education on health care. I knew, and my doctor knew, my genetic history forecast a strong possibility for a heart attack. I also knew fat, especially saturated fat, was to be avoided, and I usually did. My cholesterol was relatively low. I now realize salt is also a major heart killer. I could have done better on self-education and avoidance of salt in my already low-fat diet. I could have learned that severe persisting indigestion is also a signal of heart attack.

My learning has come the hard way. In view of my experience I am grateful to God as healer, praying friends and the excellent medical care I received. I now have a heightened awareness of the need to educate myself on recurring symptoms, and on when and how to seek assistance from medical professionals.

---

[3]Willard M. Swartley, "Mutual Aid Based in Jesus and Early Christianity," in *Building Communities of Compassion*, ed. Willard M. Swartley and Donald B. Kraybill (Scottdale, Penn.: Herald Press, 1998), pp. 21-39. See also my article "Mutual Aid," in *Dictionary of Scripture and Ethics*, ed. Joel B. Green (Grand Rapids: Baker, 2011), p. 534.

I cannot express adequately my gratitude for the prayers of many people, the wonderful care I received by the medical staff of the University of West Virginia Hospital, as well as the Rosenbaum Family House adjacent to the hospital, where after nine days of hospital care Mary and I stayed for another ten days for me to get strong enough to return to Elkhart, Indiana. What a gift also that a pilot from our congregation flew to Morgantown to take us home, while two other church men came with him to drive our car home. I received good care in my time of crisis.

Now the United States is responding to a longstanding health care challenge in which millions of people have gone without adequate care or no care at all. They lack (adequate) insurance coverage for a variety of reasons, but mostly because it is too costly or, until recently, they were excluded because of preexisting conditions. Health care costs continue to rise at an alarming rate, which forces insurance premiums to spiral. In light of Christianity's long history of providing health care (chap. 8) the church must creatively confront the issues, discerning its role in health care and health education (see chaps. 10-12). A difficult question arises: What is the church's role in relation to professional medicine and the government's role, together with health insurance companies, to cover costs?

I hope this book promotes dialogue among church people, public policymakers and health care professionals. It intends to stir the moral conscience of the church to discuss and be proactive on health education and health care issues, to continue in concern and care for the sick and dying, and to ever thank God for the healing power at work in our bodies. This book blends God's role with medical science's role in healing. It reminds us that Jesus came as God's agent of healing, and that Jesus was known as healer in his ministry on earth. The church is called to continue what Jesus began: to be a healing community. The biblical, historical, church and ethical perspectives are put in dialogue with the U.S. health care system. I consider medical, pharmaceutical and economic dimensions of health care, but leave extended treatment to others.

This book blends dual themes that I consider intrinsically related:

- health, healing and health care
- the roles of God, Jesus, Spirit and medical science in healing

The latter point is briefly but poignantly attested in a pertinent text from Sirach, a wisdom book regarded as Scripture by the Roman Catholic, Orthodox and early Anabaptist church traditions. This voice, from between the Testaments, witnesses to another perspective on healing, the role of the physician and medicine in healing. Physicians and pharmacists are recognized as allies in God's work of healing. I cite the text for its significance to a pertinent issue of our time: the relationship between God as healer and the role of medical personnel:

Honor physicians for their services,
    for the Lord created them;
for their gift of healing comes from the Most High,
    and they are rewarded by the king.
The skill of physicians makes them distinguished,
    and in the presence of the great they are admired.
The Lord created medicines out of the earth,
    and the sensible will not despise them. . . .
[The Lord] gave skill to human beings
    that he might be glorified in his marvelous works.
By them [the medicines] the physician heals and takes away pain;
    the pharmacist makes a mixture from them.
God's works will never be finished;
    and from him health spreads over all the earth.
My child, when you are ill, do not delay,
    but pray to the Lord, and he will heal you.
Give up your faults and direct your hands rightly,
    and cleanse your heart from all sin. . . .
Then give the physician his place, for the Lord created him;
    do not let him leave you, for you need him.
There may come a time when recovery lies in the hands of physicians,
    for they too pray to the Lord
that he grant them success in diagnosis
    and in healing, for the sake of preserving life.
He who sins against his Maker,
    will be defiant toward the physician. (Sir 38:1-4, 6-10, 12-15)

The text praises the skills of the physician and pharmacist.[4] But it also

[4]Frederick J. Gaiser has a splendid exposition of this text in relation to Israel's earlier emphasis on the Lord as healer. He notes that the Old Testament does not disparage physicians and then says that the Old Testament affirms both divine and human agency in healing (*Healing in the*

says, "God's works will never be finished; / and from him health [*shalom*] spreads over all the earth" (v. 8).[5] The physician is viewed as assisting God's bestowal of health. I hold this view in my own prayers and pro-active quest for health. As the progression of this book makes clear, health, healing and health care are all part of one whole. Unless the church owns these ministries, it will choose "the *hole* in our gospel" instead of the *whole* Gospel.[6]

In part one of this book I reclaim the relationship between the triune God and our healing efforts, by explicating the biblical (Old and New Testaments) understandings of health and healing.[7] In part two I focus on understanding the biblical, ethical and historical involvement of the Judeo-Christian faith in *health care* over the last three millennia. This leads to reaffirming and encouraging the synagogue's and church's mission and ministry in healing, health care and health education. In part three I connect the biblical, historical and moral perspectives with the current U.S. health care challenges.

Chapter one presents seven theses on healing, which grew out of my biblical study and the life experience of Jesus' followers. It moves toward answering the persisting question, When God does not heal me or others, what am I to believe? Chapter two focuses on health and healing as *God's* gift. It also starkly reminds us of our mortality. Chapter three focuses on Jesus' healing ministry as sign and promise of God's kingdom coming, and shows how the Christian church has regarded healing and health care as an aspect of its calling and mission, from its beginning to the present. Chapter four places the biblical study into a broader theological framework,

---

Bible: Theological Insight for Christian Ministry [Grand Rapids: Baker, 2010], p. 122). His entire chapter is most insightful, ending by reminding us that what might appear as paradoxical in both causation (including demons) and cure of illness is integrated today in African prayers for healing (ibid., pp. 117-31).

[5]Verse 15 is difficult to translate: the RSV, following the Hebrew says, "He who sins before his Maker, / may he fall into the care of a physician;" but the NRSV, following the Greek LXX, says, "He who sins against his Maker, / will be defiant toward the physician." In the RSV translation the physician is the last resort (with perhaps negative connotation). The NRSV puts God's and the physician's roles in parallel and seems to be more in keeping with what the text as a whole says.

[6]Richard Stearns, *The Hole in Our Gospel* (Nashville: Thomas Nelson, 2009).

[7]Gaiser contributes a helpful in-depth exposition of sixteen biblical stories of healing and their significance for ministry today: eight from the Old Testament, six from the new, and one on Sirach 38 and other related texts in Sirach. His final chapter blends the Testaments in his treatment of Isaiah 53:4-5.

noting the paradoxes in any theology of healing. These paradoxes guard us against pitfalls in healing ministries and acknowledge the reality of suffering. Chapter five focuses on understanding how the church's normative practices can function as healing modalities, including rituals of baptism, Eucharist, anointing with oil and more. It provides criteria to enable the church to be a healing community.

In part two, chapters six and seven examine patterns of health care in the biblical world in order to open the dialogue between biblical perspectives, including mutual aid practices and modern modalities of health care and education. Chapter eight focuses on the history of the church in healing and health care, noting that this has always been regarded as intrinsic to the church's mission. Chapter nine focuses on care for the disabled.

In part three, chapter ten describes the U.S. health care system/industry, together with the moral and economic problems it poses for sustainability. The challenges are formidable. Chapter eleven looks at health and health care in light of the biblical vision of shalom and service, and what this might mean for health care practices. Chapter twelve presents alternative philosophies and practices as models, shining lights in our present fog. The chapter narrates the vision and work of two medical doctors whose health centers provide models of holistic health care that are community oriented, focusing on those who need health care most. Health care fees are on a sliding scale, taking into account the patient's income and ability to pay. This illustrates how biblical moral priorities can be practiced in health care for those with no (or inadequate) health insurance. These models present new or renewed ways of thinking about and administering health care. They lower health care costs. The first part of the chapter addresses how U.S. health care can contain costs and foster health quality.

Appendix one describes Mennonite mission history in health care. Appendix two describes a countywide effort to provide urgent-need medical care for uninsured persons. This is a model that other faith communities may consider to replicate.

To clarify the rationale for the perspectives of this book, I identify four values that bear upon the health care system. These apply not only to the United States but worldwide:

1. *Historical learning.* Prior to the modern period, religion was the caregiver of the sick and wounded. In the West the Judeo-Christian com-

munity played a major role in health care. The church of the first three centuries did what the government of the Roman Empire did not do: risk their lives to care for the starving, save and care for babies and children left to die in the streets, and minister to those sick and dying from plagues, while even honored medical people fled to rural areas to avoid the contagion. In the fourth to eighteenth centuries the church, often allied with government, cared for the sick. Hospitals and holy places for healing developed as an arm of the church. Since the Reformation the church's involvement in health care dwindled. The Catholic Church, however, continued to be more involved in health care than Protestant churches. This was their practice historically; its involvement has roots in the Church's longstanding social teachings, based on the moral principles of the Church's faith.

One of the puzzling moral issues is, Why has the church, especially Protestant, beginning with the Reformation, largely abdicated its role in health, healing and health care? The church has sold this part of its birthright, for its healing ministry is inherent in its identity and the Great Commission. It is morally imperative to ask, How can the church reclaim its calling to be healer in the context of present-day health education needs and prevailing health care endeavors?

2. Mission perspectives. In the nineteenth century, Christianity's missionary impulse was impelled by its commitment to literacy, education and health care services. Health care was an integral part of the gospel. Medical missions, begun around 1860, gradually extended medical services into almost every known country of the world, including newly known tribal groups (chap. 8). Historically, health care was integral to Christianity's and Judaism's moral vision. I am not arguing that church or faith-based organizations should take over the government's responsibility for health care. In our pluralistic society that would not work. But we need to recover churchly concern and action for health care that includes the poor and sick that *most need* medical treatment.

3. Theological considerations. God's desire, according to Scripture, is shalom for all people. *Shalom* is often defined as "wholeness" in physical health and communal relationships. *Shalom* includes a person's physical, emotional and mental welfare. When some people are deprived of health care, communal shalom is threatened.

4. Moral/ethical issues. The present complex U.S. health care system faces us with difficult moral challenges. The cost of health insurance is so high that unemployed and poor people generally cannot afford it. Because health care is at the mercy of market profit by numerous "players" in the system, Mary McDonough aptly titles her book *Can a Health Care Market Be Moral?* Whatever position we take on health care reform, we must ask what our moral priorities are. Do we think only of ourselves and the needs of people most like us, or do we try to think as Jesus thought: How can the sick and those who desperately need healing and health care in our society find it? What is our moral passion on this issue that has reached crisis proportion in the economy and social welfare of the United States? And why?

This book does not address adequately the more technical issues of funding health care, although it does present some alternative models to the dominant form of health care in the United States. Experts in the fields of finance and researchers in health care delivery systems have and will continue to address those areas. This book's contribution is from the perspective of biblical, ecclesial and moral passion and precedent. Health care is a moral priority, as the number of the underinsured and uninsured continues to rise. The complexity of U.S. health care has to a significant extent paralyzed providers in their ability to render their services well at a sustainable cost. At the same time, the cost of services rendered and technologies utilized plays into the system's unsustainable future. Perhaps we can learn from other national health care systems, as T. R. Reid did in his international quest to learn how eight different national health care systems work and what each would do to cure his lame shoulder. The United States' answer was a shoulder replacement but other countries had other solutions at varied costs.[8] Most interesting!

---

[8]T. R. Reid, *The Healing of America: A Global Quest for Better, Cheaper, and Fairer Health Care* (New York: Penguin Press, 2009). Taiwan and Switzerland are most interesting and one or the other may be predictive of health care's future in the United States (ibid., pp. 164-81)! Reid describes Japan's efficient health care system as "Bismarck [Germany's system] on Rice" (ibid., pp. 82-102). Canada's is "Sorry to Keep You Waiting" (ibid., pp. 125-41).

PART ONE

Healing

1

❖

Seven Theses

FROM SCRIPTURE TO TODAY

Teach me your way, O LORD,
that I may walk in your truth;
give me an undivided heart to revere your name.

Psalm 86:11

Who can tell what a day may bring forth?
Cause me, therefore, gracious God
to live every day as if it were to be my last,
for I know not but that it may be such.
Cause me to live now as I shall wish
I had done when I come to die.

Thomas À Kempis, The Imitation of Christ

Any topic or issue must be addressed from the context of a larger biblical theology. Both this chapter and the next four try to do just that—to forge a path toward a biblical theology of healing. Chapters two and three focus on the Old and New Testaments, respectively. In chapter four I examine four biblical-theological paradoxes that are foundational to understand healing. Chapter five views the church as a healing community.

To grasp the full range of the healing emphases in Scripture, a trinitarian view is helpful, since each person of the Trinity is portrayed in Christian Scripture with healing emphases. For example, in brief:

God as healer.

Bless the LORD, O my soul,
 and do not forget all his benefits—
who forgives all your iniquity,
 who heals all your diseases,
who redeems your life from the Pit,
 who crowns you with steadfast love and mercy. (Ps 103:2-4)

This psalm is one of many that acknowledge God as healer of disease (cf. Ex 15:26). Not until later in Israel's history were the gifts of medicine and pharmacy also acknowledged as beneficial to healing (see Sir 38).

Jesus as healer. After Jesus healed the Roman centurion's servant by speaking the word of healing from a distance, Matthew reports an evening healing event:

> They brought to him many who were possessed with demons; and he cast out the spirits with a word, and cured all who were sick. This was to fulfill what had been spoken through the prophet Isaiah, "He took our infirmities and bore our diseases." (Mt 8:16-17)

Chapter three shows how integral Jesus' healing ministry was to his mission. Healing and salvation are closely linked. This text unites Jesus' healing with his exorcisms and sees both as the fulfillment of Isaiah's prophecy.

Holy Spirit as healer.

> I consider that the sufferings of this present time are not worth comparing with the glory about to be revealed to us. For the creation waits with eager longing for the revealing of the children of God; for the creation was subjected to futility, not of its own will but by the will of the one who subjected it, in hope that the creation itself will be set free from its bondage to decay and will obtain the freedom of the glory of the children of God. We know that the whole creation has been groaning in labor pains until now; and not only the creation, but we ourselves, who have the first fruits of the Spirit, groan inwardly while we wait for adoption, the redemption of our bodies. For in hope we were saved. Now hope that is seen is not hope. For who hopes for what is seen? But if we hope for what we do not see, we wait for it with patience.
>
> Likewise the Spirit helps us in our weakness; for we do not know how to pray as we ought, but that very Spirit intercedes with sighs too deep for

words. And God, who searches the heart, knows what is the mind of the Spirit, because the Spirit intercedes for the saints according to the will of God. (Rom 8:18-27)

The Holy Spirit as healer complements God as healer and Jesus as healer. The Spirit reminds us that though we now enjoy redemption's first-fruits, more is to come. Our bodies, medically and miraculously healed at times, waste away, but the Spirit-cry within us, *Abba*, promises redemption of our bodies when we are released from our present groaning. Our dying is transformed into life with the triune God eternally.

Further, the Spirit is our intercessor when we don't know what to pray for, or we are so heavily burdened we cannot find words to pray. The Spirit takes our groans and translates them into petitions to God and Jesus for our good outcome. The Spirit also comforts us and assures us "all is well." We can rest in our groaning and trust the Spirit to present the right healing prayer to God.

Within this trinitarian context I propose seven theses on healing:

Thesis 1. God intends shalom and community for humans and all creation, but sin and Satan play adversarial roles against us and against God's intentions for us.

We live in a marvelous, mysterious world created by God. Whether we are enraptured by endless space with its billions of galaxies or the incomprehensible intricacies of our DNA codes, we know this world has been created by an almighty God. More than two hundred billion stars light the night sky of our Milky Way galaxy. But the human being is also a great wonder of wonders, with DNA codes and brains of incomprehensible complexity: "the number of synaptic interconnections in a single human brain vastly exceeds the number of stars in our Milky Way: 10^{15} synapses versus about 10^{11} stars."[1] Living in this vast universe with another hundred billion galaxies beyond our Milky Way, we experience daily delights to the eye, ear, smell, taste and touch. When life is functioning normally, we say, "Yes, this is a good world." When all is well, we call it health, and we claim it as a gift from God.

But then, as it does for most at some time, illness strikes, with a variety of faces. We wonder if God Almighty has abandoned us. We pray for

---

[1]Owen Gingerich, *God's Universe* (Cambridge, Mass.: Belknap Press of Harvard University Press, 2006), p. 30.

healing, but sometimes don't know how to pray. Sometimes our prayers are miraculously answered, but often not, at least in the way we would like. We then doubt God's good world, and we wonder who else besides God is playing in this drama of history, obstructing the shalom of our health.

The Scriptures reassure us that, yes, God created us, and the creation is good, but another power, an adversary against God, is also part of the historical stage. On the one hand, we humans are created in the "image of God," with the capacity and desire for human relationships (i.e., community) and capability to exercise dominion over all creation. This is the cultural mandate and opportunity, involving work, creative invention, managing, preserving and tending (Gen 2:15). Community and dominion (tending creation) are essential components of health. When we become ill, we feel incapacitated, precisely in our freedom to exercise these innate, God-given capacities.

But the biblical analysis goes deeper. It tells us there is a primal and ontological reason why the good creation, and our experience of it, is marred. Incited by the tempter, the snake, indeed the devil (Wis 2:24; Rev 12:9), our first set of parents yielded to the desire to be as God, thereby gaining the ability to know both good and evil. Rather than relating only to God in a trustful relationship, humans chose to obey the voice of the snake. In biblical thought post-Genesis 3, the creation is flawed and fallen as the result of this human opening to the evil power that works against God and God's good creation. For this reason Paul writes in Romans 8:18-22 that the whole creation, which was subjected to futility, will be set free one day. Thus with all of creation, *we* also groan while we wait for adoption, the redemption of our bodies.

Precisely within this context God reaches out to us in grace and helpful provision. God gives laws, the Ten Commandments, to enable humans to experience a goodness approximating the intention of creation, living together in shalom. Each of the Ten Commandments contributes to the health of the community. Breaking any one of them jeopardizes the health and welfare of the community.

Individualism is one of the greatest threats to community health. One person's violation of the operative rules of community life affects the whole community's health and relation to God. Rampant in Western society, individualism has had a disastrous effect upon community well-being.

Our modern world highly values individual choice and self-fulfillment—and both are "good" within limitations. When pursued without regard for community life, the quest to freely choose whatever we desire stifles communal shalom. This is shockingly evident in the economic meltdown of 2008-2011, where greed and corruption in high places with unregulated free enterprise, ruined corporate welfare in the United States and globally. In turn, this negatively affects the community's shalom-health (unemployment, foreclosures and bankruptcies). The twenty-two-day war from Christmas 2008 to January 18, 2009, between Israel and the Gaza Palestinians caused horrific destruction of shalom. Embargoes denying entrance of food and medicines into Gaza, or into any country, as was the case in Iraq for years and now Iran, destroy a people's shalom. Without laws for community life, and security from marauding neighbors, the shalom welfare of any community is quickly undermined. For this reason God gave to Israel not only the Ten Commandments but also a system of built-in checks against human greed and corruption. The system of sabbath, sabbaticals and Jubilee celebrates equality, even between slaves and masters, instituting forgiveness of debts and release to the slaves every seven years, and redistribution of land and wealth every fifty years, in the year of Jubilee. The seventh year sabbatical also restores the corporate welfare of the people through its mandatory forgiveness of debts, release of slaves who desired release, and giving the land a year of rest, thus regenerating its productivity. Because Israel did not keep these laws, God punished them with exile (Ex 31:12-17; Deut 5:12-15; Is 56:1-2; 58:1-9, 13-14; Jer 32; cf. Mal 2:4-9).

Health is a spiritual issue.[2] When we fail to live in harmony with God's design for human community, we aid and abet the powers of illness in our bodies and minds. Of crucial importance here is the role of repentance, confession and forgiveness in the structure of a community's life. We are all sinners and we will all make choices at some time that cause pain and psychic stress to ourselves and others. The key for people's health is whether these wrongs and hurts can be healed through forgiveness and mutual care for one another even in the midst of health tragedies. This

---

[2]See Harold G. Koenig, *Medicine, Religion And Health: Where Science and Spirituality Meet* (West Conshohocken, Penn.: Templeton Foundation Press, 2008), and James Lapsley, *Salvation and Health: The Interlocking Process of Life* (Philadelphia: Westminster Press, 1972).

theme, like many others, reminds us all that we live by God's grace shed abroad in our hearts through the Holy Spirit, who gives us hope amid adversity (Rom 5:3-5).

Thesis 2. God is God and we are weak, mortal and frail creatures (Ps 49; 103).

Another part of biblical creation theology is that humans are *adam*, made from the ground (*adamah*), and are thus frail, mortal creatures. This means our health is linked to the earth and our care for it. Otherwise we curse the ground from which we have come and on which our health depends, in food, living space and aesthetic beauty. Also our relation to the earth reminds us that we need to accept our mortality and finitude. Wanting to be "like God" and thus denying or evading our mortality continues the Fall. Arising from human disobedience, it fails to let God be God and to let humans accept their creaturely dependence on God as Creator. Accepting our creature identity is an essential part of human health.

Even though animated by God's breathing his spirit into a dusty art form—the human body—to become living souls (*nephesh*), we are still needy, vulnerable people, dependent on God's sustaining presence and power. We must begin by emphasizing our human frailty, thus avoiding an easy, shallow optimism and unrealistic appraisal of the human situation (see chap. 2). This is the duality of our human nature: constrained by mortality and yet by God's life-giving Spirit, we surge from one degree of understanding, discovery and invention to another. Finitude and freedom coexist in our being.[3]

Many times the Psalms emphasize the frailty of our human existence (e.g., 90; 103). In Psalm 39 the psalmist cries to God, saying, "how fleeting my life is." I am only a "passing guest, an alien, like all my forebears."

Thesis 3. Illness puts us in a quandary before God, for it interrupts and challenges God's good world in personal experience. The Psalms lead us in voicing our cries of lament to God.

The lament psalms are cries of the righteous, appealing to God for healing, at least to be mindful of the desolate, lonely feeling of the human condition. Psalms 6, 30, and 88 are especially relevant. Psalm 30 specifically describes the sick person's loss of shalom, interrupted by some type of

---

[3]Cf. Gilbert Meilaender, introduction to *Biothethics: A Primer for Christians* (Grand Rapids: Eerdmans, 1996), pp. 3-4.

illness. Psalm 30 traverses three stages of experience: original shalom (v. 6), the disorientation of sickness and cry for help and healing (vv. 2, 8-10), and restoration to life in which "you have turned my mourning into dancing" so "that my soul may praise you and not be silent. O Lord my God, I will give thanks to you forever" (vv. 3, 11-12).

Numerous images describe the distress of the sufferer: troubled bones, no soundness of flesh, eyes wasting from grief, wounds grow foul and fester, heart hot within, I mire in the waters, the floods overwhelm me. In many of these images a sense of sinking and being overwhelmed by chaos emerges. The evils of sickness and death are part of the chaos that Yahweh's divine power holds back from swooping in and down upon life.

Psalm 88, similar to much of Psalm 22, expresses the human sense of Godforsakenness. It likely is describing the feeling of one mentally ill. Though it begins with an appeal to God to hear his cry (vv. 1-2), it dwells on the troubles of the sufferer. The psalmist feels forsaken, shunned by his companions, sinking down to the pit, abandoned to *Abaddon*—the place of darkness. The psalm never turns the corner to praise God, as most of the lament psalms do.

Martin Marty tells how he wanted to skip Psalm 88 as it came up in the daily reading schedule he and his wife followed daily. This scheduled psalm came up at the time she was dying of cancer. He began reading another psalm, but his wife stopped him, asking, "Why *not* read Psalm 88?" He told her it didn't turn the corner to praise. She insisted he read it anyway, since it gave voice to her (and likely also his) feelings. Scripture in its diversity connects with the range of our human experience, and illness is no exception. In this case, it voices the anguish of the soul.

Psalm 103, in contrast, is a jubilant song of thanksgiving for healing, voicing the experience of illness and recovery that deepened appreciation for God's mighty works of salvation and steadfast love. The sufferer is restored to where he or she can again praise God, function freely in the community, and thus reclaim shalom.

Thesis 4. Suffering means not divine absence but testing, even God's love for us. In our suffering God is not absent but present in love (the theodicy question is addressed more fully in chap. 4).

We hear briefly four voices from Scripture: Jeremiah, Habakkuk, Isaiah and Job.

Jeremiah, more than any other prophet, writes about the loss of shalom
and healing for the nation:

> We look for peace [*shalom*], but find no good,
> for a time of healing [*marpe*], but there is terror instead. (Jer 8:15; cf. Jer 14:19)

Jeremiah scores Israel's leaders for only a shalom-healing veneer: the
priest and the prophets have "treated the wound of my people carelessly,
saying, 'Peace, peace,' when there is no peace" (Jer 8:11; 6:14). Hence Jeremiah's "grief is beyond healing" (Jer 8:18 RSV); there is "no balm in
Gilead" and "no physician there . . . the health of my poor people [has] not
been restored" (Jer 8:22).

In his "Confessions" Jeremiah cries out for personal healing, linked to
the nation's shalom and healing:

> Heal me, O LORD, and I shall be healed;
> save me, and I shall be saved;
> for you are my praise. (Jer 17:14)

Jeremiah as prophet of pathos, like Hosea, embodies the sickness and
no-shalom health of the nation. Jeremiah laments the lack of and need for
shalom and healing for himself and the nation.[4] As Joseph Savage sum-
marizes Jeremiah's frequent linkage of shalom and healing: "Where a
fracturing of shalom is evidenced, there is simultaneously a fracturing of
health/healing and vice versa; . . . the terms of *shalom* and health/healing
are mutually inclusive; one cannot be had without the other."[5] From Jeremiah we learn that all sufferers are not sinners; *some are suffering saints*
because of the nation's transgression.

Habakkuk is plagued with the question of why the wicked prosper (a
form of shalom) and overtake the righteous, "so that justice goes forth
perverted" (Hab 1:4 RSV). The answer he receives, after he takes his stand
to watch, wait and listen, is that "the righteous live by their faith" (Hab
2:4). He then reaffirms faith that "the earth will be filled with the
knowledge of the glory of the LORD as the waters cover the sea" (Hab

---

[4]For an extensive study of Jeremiah's dual use of shalom for peace and healing (often for the nation) see Joseph M. Savage, "Shalom and Its Relationship to Health/Healing in the Hebrew
Scriptures: A Contextual and Semantic Study of the Books of Psalms and Jeremiah" (Ph.D.
diss., Florida State University, 2001), pp. 105-214.
[5]Ibid., p. 213.

2:14). Climactically, he sees "the LORD . . . in his holy temple; let all the earth keep silence before him" (Hab 2:20). From his voice we learn that *some sufferers are worshiping saints.*

Isaiah's "servant of the Lord" lost his shalom through the horrible desolation of exile as a nation. Lamenting for Jerusalem (cornerstone of shalom) by the waters of Babylon (Ps 137), God reveals to him proclamation of the gospel of peace (Is 52:7), a word of hope in the midst of the suffering. Notably, the wounds of the servant, suffering in the cause of God's justice (Is 42:1-4), are the means of shalom and healing for many (Is 53:5-12). In this we learn that *a sufferer can also be a savior.*

Job's witness, arising from within the wisdom tradition itself, plumbs the depths of the sufferer's agony and quest for meaning to suffering. He accepts part of the conventional answer: God is to be addressed as responsible for suffering. Job also tempers this judgment in that he realizes Satan also plays a role in suffering, though still under God's sovereignty (cf. Is 45:7). But he does not accept the other part of the conventional wisdom represented by his friends: that suffering is just punishment for sin and guilt. He cries out for someone to listen to him and present the indictment so he can refute it step by step (Job 31:35-37). He knows he is righteous and the cause of his affliction lies not in his sin and guilt. The way (*derek*) out of his prison comes by an unlocking from the outside; God answers through the whirlwind: humans cannot presume to know the ways of God; in the midst of suffering God is still there;[6] and *the righteous sufferer is a friend of God.*

On the one hand, sickness and suffering appear to fight against God, to be of the devil, but Scripture also frames suffering differently. God hears the cry of the sufferer and, as loving God, is present in suffering, in Christ's and in ours (more in chap. 5). Meilaender addresses this early on in his treatment of bioethics. I sum it up in three points:

- At the heart of Christian belief lies a suffering, crucified God.

- Suffering is not a good thing, not something one ought to seek for oneself or others.

- *But it is an evil out of which God, revealed in the crucified and risen Jesus, can bring good. We must therefore always be of two minds about it.*[7]

[6]Klaus Seybold and Ulrich B. Mueller, *Sickness and Healing*, trans. Douglas W. Stott (Nashville: Abingdon, 1978), p. 81.
[7]Meilaender, *Bioethics*, pp. 7-8.

Thesis 5. Jesus is Healer-Savior and leads us in faith and prayer.

In the Gospels healings of various types were an essential part of Jesus' mission (developed in chap. 3). From Jesus' compassion and healings a new community emerged, those who followed Jesus, both women and men (Lk 8:1-3; 9:1-4). Love and healing go hand in hand. As C. S. Lewis puts it in *Shadowlands*, "We love, to know we are not alone." The bond that unites Jesus and his followers is that they—indeed, we—have been touched with love and healed. Love, healing and peace are a seamless garment.

In Jesus' healings *faith* (either that of the sick person or of friends, as in Mk 2:5) often plays a significant role in the healing, but not in exorcisms or in all healings, as, for example, the healing of the man born blind in John 9 or raising the widow's son at Nain (Lk 7:11-17, though it generated faith). This raises the issue of Jesus healings as "faith healings."[8] Because our modern conceptions of the relation between the physical/material and spiritual worlds do not mesh well with the worldview of the first century, the matter is complex. It is further complicated by the Calvinist and Arminian differences over the origin and nature of faith. If faith is seen as an act of the human will, which can be conjured up by our efforts, then no, the healings are not faith healings. If faith is seen as gift of God apart from the gospel message awakening faith, then no, also, the healings are not faith healings. But if faith is seen as openness to divine presence in humble reliant trust, then, yes, these are faith healings. For then people respond to Jesus as the one who mediates the divine power to heal. But unbelief constrains Jesus' healing as in Nazareth where people regarded him as only the son of Joseph and Mary. But even then there's a curious mix of can't and can: "And he could do no deed of power there, except that he laid his hands on a few sick people and cured them" (Mk 6:5). *Faith* and healing occur more normatively when people accept Jesus as messianic revealer of the kingdom. In every age the church needs to test whether claims to faith healing are fact or fraud. Ted Schwartz sees this as a continuing challenge and task for the church.[9]

---

[8]For a helpful discussion of the faith issue, see Francis MacNutt, *Healing* (Notre Dame, Ind.: Ave Maria Press, 1999), pp. 89-105. A related issue is the "if it is your will" condition when praying for healing. It is better to change "if" to "according to your will and purpose." Cf. the prayer suggested by Darryl Zoller, "The Ministry of Christian Healing," *Sharing the Practice* 28, no. 1 (Winter 2005): 4.
[9]Ted Schwartz, *Healing in the Name of God: Faith or Fraud?* (Grand Rapids: Zondervan, 1993).

How do we value and assess miracles as an ongoing ministry of the church? Scripture does not promise that miracles occur in accord with some formula of human faith. Rather, miracles are *given* as bestowals of the kingdom's presence exalting Jesus Christ.[10] For those whose views of reality are not fenced by rationalistic walls that separate the material from the spiritual,[11] an openness to the presence of the spiritual may and, because God is gracious, likely will be answered by special signs of the kingdom—wonders, mighty works, call them miracles if you will—which unmistakably extol Jesus Christ as God's mender of groaning creation. Prayer, inspired by Spirit power and in the name of Jesus, connects us to the God from whom all healing blessings flow. Hence prayer is essential, providing openness to God's healing of sickness as sign of kingdom presence. Prayer also provides the empowerment to endure suffering in the hope of the ultimate healing, and prayer paradoxically also enables healing. (As I edit this, I marvel at a "miracle" reported this past Sunday and more fully in today's e-mail: a woman in her early eighties and last days of life, all thought, inexplicably rallied and is now living toward robust life again! The doctors have no explanation.)

In Luke 10 Jesus' healing ministry continues in the mission of the Seventy. Healing is linked to two other major themes of the Gospel: the coming of the kingdom of God and the downfall of Satan. Further, the gospel of peace is the greeting that elicits receptivity or rejection. Receptivity and faith in response to the gospel of peace are crucial. How do we hear the good news Isaiah prophesied: "How beautiful upon the mountains are the feet of the messenger who announces peace" (Is 52:7)? Jesus' entire ministry is summed by his "preaching the good news (i.e., gospel) of peace . . . and healing all that were oppressed . . . doing good and healing all those oppressed by the devil" (Acts 10:36, 38 RSV; see fig. 3.1).

Jesus' compassion, his access policy and people's faith are significant features in Jesus' healings. These are interconnected with Jesus' messianic

---

[10]This is the emphasis in Howard M. Ervin, *Healing: Sign of the Kingdom* (Peabody, Mass.: Hendrickson, 2002).

[11]From a post-Kantian rationalist view, any reported miraculous healing will first be assessed by the empirical standards of previously observed phenomena, on which basis a claim of a *unique* healing will be doubted. Or, if one's philosophical inclination is more global, accepting religious beliefs in spirit powers, the miracle claim will be judged to be magic by an unbeliever, as the pagan philosopher Celsus judged healing miracles by Christians in the second century.

mission: to bring near God's reign of goodness and wholeness on earth, and to drive back the powers of Satan and sin, evil and darkness. Proclaiming God's reign in Luke is announcing the good news of peace (fulfilling Is 52:7; see chap. 3). Further, however, as Michael Brown points out, "these supernatural healings were not merely authenticating signs of his divinity or messiahship; . . . rather, they reflected the very heart of God toward sick and suffering humanity."[12] This balance of emphases is important in constructing a theology of healing in the life of the church today.

Thesis 6. The Spirit too is healer and is the divine pledge of complete healing.

A key New Testament perspective is that believers share in the sufferings of the present eon. Indeed, all creation has been groaning, waiting—standing on tiptoe—with eager longing for God's final redeeming, healing work on behalf of those holding this Christian hope. God's children await the redemption of their bodies (Rom 8:18-23), which correlates with God's defeat of the last enemy, death (1 Cor 15:26, 57-58). The redemption of the body is based on the central Christian belief of Jesus' resurrection from the dead. Hence, in uniting with Christ's death and resurrection in baptism, believers receive the *arrabon*, the Holy Spirit, as down payment for the final redemption, resurrection in the life to come.

As long as this temporal tension is a part of our salvation, we share in the groaning and sufferings of "waiting in hope." As Christiaan Beker says:

> For in their own bodies, Christians live existentially the tension of their present uncompleted existence in solidarity with an unredeemed creation, and they must therefore yearn for the consummation of the resurrection, which is nothing but God's triumph over the power of death that poisons his creation.[13]

From this perspective of suffering and hope we encounter distinctive features of a Christian approach to health: Christ's work is viewed as a mending of all creation so that our personal health is seen within that larger context. The gift of the Spirit is our experiential participation in the overlap of the ages. It is a source of empowerment from the standpoint of God's final healing of all things (*ta panta*). Kenneth Bakken emphasizes these points:

---

[12]Michael L. Brown, *Israel's Divine Healer* (Grand Rapids: Zondervan, 1995), p. 222.
[13]J. Christiaan Beker, *Suffering and Hope: The Biblical Vision and the Human Predicament* (Grand Rapids: Eerdmans, 1994), p. 17.

God brings us health in many forms, but until we are touched by the reality of the Spirit, we cannot be truly whole. Our spiritual life, then, becomes a key factor in our journey toward wholeness. Krister Stendahl, former dean of the Harvard Divinity School, has said that God's agenda is the mending of creation. God is active in creation and is present in us—for our healing and ultimate salvation. The word *salvation*, from the root word *salvus*, means "healed." Thus, an abundant life of wholeness comes only in the mending, the healing.[14]

Thesis 7. The church is called to be God's face of healing in this world. Our mission is to mediate the healing power of God, Christ, Holy Spirit through prayer and exercise of faith.

In *Practicing Theology*, Tammy Williams insightfully develops a threefold analysis of practices of healing in African American churches. She assesses three streams of healing practice (see table 1.1).[15]

Table 1.1. Summary of Three Streams of Healing Practice

Type	Which Churches?	Action	Strength	Weakness
Traditional	Mainline	Caring	God is free: heal or not. Incarnates God's love	Gives sense: God okays sickness; God's will, some are sick = "cross"
"Word of faith"	Pentecostal	Cure	God is faithful/will heal Jesus is doctor	Sickness suggests weak faith, spirituality, and excludes some
"Holistic"	Many churches	Healing	Takes account of culture, community; preventive	Weak in beliefs about healing Little is said about God

While table 1.1 does not do justice to the many good points developed in Williams's article (she begins her discussion of each type with a "gospel song" text), it does show a profile of difference, found not only in African

[14]Kenneth L. Bakken, *The Call to Wholeness: Health as Spiritual Journey* (New York: Crossroad, 1985), p. 46.
[15]Tammy Williams, "Is There a Doctor in the House?" in *Practicing Theology: Beliefs and Practices in Christian Life*, ed. Miroslav Volf and Dorothy C. Bass (Grand Rapids: Eerdmans, 2002), pp. 94-120. Williams rightly points out that this is true of some Pentecostals, but not nearly all. Many fall into the more traditional type, and more and more lean toward the "holistic" type.

American churches but in churches generally. In introducing her article, she makes an important point, "Because healing is often practiced at the edge of life and death and often involves persons who are very vulnerable, it is essential that practitioners understand what they are actually doing and why they are doing it."[16] While Williams leans toward the "holistic" type, she affirms elements in each and candidly identifies the dangers and weaknesses in each. She ends her article with a section titled "There Is a Doctor in the House and Jesus Is His Name," answering the question in the title of her article. She calls for solidarity with those ill, emphasizes the need for spiritual transformation even though cure or recovery may not occur, and that doctor Jesus' "aim is not to cure and then disappear but whose healing more profoundly consists in our knowledge of him and his presence with us. . . . [T]he aim of healing is 'getting to know the doctor better' and honoring our relationship to him in 'sickness and in health,' in 'life and death' (Phil 1:20)."[17]

HERMENEUTICAL REFLECTIONS

1. I've endeavored to outline a biblical theology of health and sickness as a context to understand the biblical claim that God is healer, Jesus Christ is healer and the Holy Spirit is healer. It is important to put these theses in dialogue with the entire sweep of Scripture (see chap. 4). Similarly, it is helpful to consider crosscultural perspectives, especially as we are more and more in dialogue with cultures other than our own in the church's mission. In some cultures emphasis falls on miraculous healing, including exorcism of evil spirits. The setting in which one lives and serves generally determines the emphasis. This does not change our basic beliefs in God's good creation, the reality of fallen nature due to human sin, and God's saving and healing action set forth in biblical revelation, culminating in Jesus Christ.

A pertinent critique may come from medical personnel: "You have not dealt adequately with the relation between modern scientific and biblical understandings of healing. While you noted Sirach 38 that holds the two together, we know so much more now than we did two thousand years ago, and we can now accomplish many more cures through medical

---

[16]Ibid., p. 96.
[17]Ibid., p. 120.

means." This is true. We gratefully acknowledge that medical advances and expertise now can cure many illnesses and thus contribute to healing.

Sometimes a distinction is made between *curing* and *healing*. *Curing* is the medical gift and *healing* is God's gift through believers praying for Jesus Christ to heal.[18] Thus a person may be cured of an illness or disease, but underlying causative stress, distress or even sin may not be healed. But I think this distinction does not stand. The NRSV, apparently influenced by this distinction in health and healing literature, translates *therapeuō* in Matthew 9:35; 10:1, 8; and Luke 10:9; for example, as "cure(ing)" and *iaomai* in Luke 6:18-19 and Acts 10:38, for example, as "heal(ing)."[19] Thus Jesus was miracle healer and doctor curer. This distinction, however, becomes problematic in current everyday usage. For my own situation I would need to say I was healed, at least in some respects, but not completely cured. But it would be just as true to say I was cured, at least in part, but not completely healed. Theologically, healing is complete only when we are redeemed from these mortal bodies and given a spiritual body— difficult indeed to conceive (1 Cor 15:42-49)—in the resurrection at the last day (Jn 6:39-40, 44, 54). It makes more sense to say medical expertise does its best to cure illness and thereby contributes to healing. Conversely, when we pray for healing, we hope for cure. We acknowledge too that we may experience aspects of healing (emotional and spiritual) without a physical cure. Many of us live with illness of one sort or another; we are neither completely cured nor healed. But as Christian believers we expect some day to be completely healed. Healing is a broader category than curing. Curing stands in the service of healing.

2. A second hermeneutical reflection focuses on how well this approach fits the three "focal images" that Richard Hays has proposed as normative criteria in his ethical study of the New Testament.[20] To what extent does this analysis fit the moral priorities of *community*, *cross* and *new creation*? *Community* is integral to the basic definition given to health and illness—

---

[18]One might see articles in church papers titled "Healed, But Not Cured." The point is good, but it does not resolve the relation between curing and healing.

[19]One might appeal to key Bible dictionaries or lexicons for this distinction, but it does not hold in all cases. In BAGD *therapeuō* meaning #2 has "care for . . . treat (medically), to heal, restore" (*cure* is not used). In 2 Clement 9:7 God is the *therapeuōn*, the healer.

[20]Richard B. Hays, *The Moral Vision of the New Testament: Community, Cross, New Creation* (San Francisco: HarperSanFrancisco, 1996), pp. 193-206.

the experience or absence of shalom. In both Testaments illness jeopardizes community. It may be the result of conflicts in the community, as Paul declares regarding the eating patterns at the sacred meal in Corinth (1 Cor 11:17-22, 27-34): "For this reason many of you are weak and ill, and some have died" (v. 30). In the healing stories of Jesus, healing restored the person to full life in the community. Indeed, the biblical way of viewing illness and wellness is much more community dependent than are our modern ways. Regarding *cross*, it is not difficult to see an analogical connection between the human sufferer during illness and Jesus' suffering on the cross, even though the significance and intensity of the two types of suffering are different. Both illness and cross confront us with the misery and mystery of suffering. Thesis four speaks of suffering in sickness as a type of cross experience. Like the cross, it calls us to trust God when the sun does not shine, when foes oppress us and when we don't feel like praying. Chapters four and nine treat the role of the cross more explicitly. *Cross* also figures into chapter five as a theological symbol or image that carries healing power.

Regarding *new creation*, the treatment contributes much. The emphasis on Romans 8 and the role of the Holy Spirit guard against superclaims, false claims and deceptive reliance on easy formulas: "If you believe enough you will be cured." I affirm full and ultimate healing, but in the new creation, when we receive new redeemed bodies.

3. The treatment of this topic falls mostly into two of Hays's *modes* of moral appeal: paradigms and symbolic worldview.[21] The paradigms are the stories of sickness and healing in both Testaments. These contribute basic theological perspectives.[22] Descriptions of the human predicament and affirmation of resurrection hope provide the fundamental theological categories for understanding the tension between God's good created world and illness we humans experience. They are part and parcel of the symbolic world of Scripture: Genesis 1–3; the Gospel stories of healing, set within the context of Jesus proclaiming God's reign; and Romans 8:18-39 describe the symbolic world of the larger scriptural narrative in its

---

[21]Ibid., pp. 208-9.

[22]Frederick Gaiser's intensive study of sixteen biblical healing narratives and his "summary" is most helpful. This book's scope is broader. See Frederick Gaiser, *Healing in the Bible: Theological Insights for Christian Ministry* (Grand Rapids: Baker Academic, 2010), pp. 239-50.

testimony to God, Jesus Christ and Holy Spirit as healer.

4. Whether the interpretation stands in the service of obedience to and worship of God is a critical test. When ill and dying, I would hope I could write as my brother did. In my own experience I meditated on some precious verse or theme from each psalm—as many as I could—and discovered that, with my mind uncluttered from duties, deadlines and worries, the psalms led me into communion with my holy, loving heavenly *Abba*.

2

❖

Healing in the Old Testament

I am the LORD who heals you.

Exodus 15:26

Israel viewed God the Lord as its healer, both of physical and spiritual sickness.[1] Seeking help from physicians was viewed negatively (2 Chron 16:12; Job 13:4; Jer 8:22ff.),[2] though later in Sirach (c. 200 B.C.) the contributions of physicians and medicine are valued (see Sir 38).[3]

Given our contemporary world, we know that medical skill and pharmaceuticals play a major role in curing sickness and disease. In this chapter I focus primarily on the Old Testament and especially on the Psalms, which were Jesus' Scripture and that of the early church. Both Testaments present significant insights on healing. The Old Testament is precondition

---

[1]The most thorough study of healing in the Old Testament is Michael L. Brown's *Israel's Divine Healer* (Grand Rapids: Zondervan, 1995). Similarly, the most thorough treatment of the Bible and healing is by medical doctor and theologian John Wilkinson, *The Bible and Healing: A Medical and Theological Commentary* (Grand Rapids: Eerdmans, 1998). For wider scope of treatment, see Morton Kelsey, *Healing and Christianity* (Minneapolis: Augsburg, 1995). Allen Verhey highlights the "strangeness" of the world of healing in the Old Testament in that both Israel's sin and God's wrath often function as direct explanation, even judgment, for personal sickness or a communitywide plague. Nonetheless, he says health is not the main focus, but healing and health stand in the service of God's blessing and covenant faithfulness, culminating in Jesus ("Health and Healing in Memory of Jesus," in Health and Healing, *Ex Auditu* 21 [2005]: 31-41). For wider treatment of sickness and healing, see his 2002 and 2003 entries in the bibliography.

[2]Howard Clark Kee, "Medicine and Healing," in *Anchor Bible Dictionary*, ed. David Noel Freedman et al. (New York: Doubleday, 1992), 4:660.

[3]Judeo-Christian faith is not the only religion in which divine power is believed available for healing. Many traditional societies look to the local shaman (or "witch doctor") for healing. Eastern religions too promise healing, with alternative medical procedures (see the excursus at the end of this chapter).

for the New. The *New* Testament can be adequately understood only through the lens of the Old, as Jesus himself and the early church understood the Scriptures.[4] Since God the Lord is healer in the Old Testament, we rightly expect Jesus to be healer in the New Testament.

Two related convictions are foundational to biblical faith. First, as humans we are mortal in nature. Second, the Lord God is our Creator-Sustainer-Healer. We must own our mortality, lest with sophisticated technology and medical advances to extend life we are prone to forget this.

OWNING OUR MORTALITY

In his article "Human Wholeness in Biblical Perspective," Waldemar Janzen contends that Christians too often wrongly begin their understanding of human nature with the emphasis that we are created in God's image. This, he argues, can too easily lead to a shallow optimism and unrealistic appraisal of the human situation. Rather, he emphasizes the need to begin with an awareness of human frailty. He reminds us that the Genesis narratives emphasize that humans are *adam*, taken from the ground, *adamah* (Gen 1:27; 2:7). God says to the first human pair, "You are dust, and to dust you shall return" (Gen 3:19). Even though animated by the divine breath, the human is only a living *nephesh*, which may be translated "desire, soul, life, person, self." However, its basic meaning is "throat, neck." Hence humans are "all throat" (compare "all thumbs"). As if this is not enough to underscore our frailty and finitude, humans are designated by another word some 150 times, the word *basar* meaning "flesh." Flesh designates human weakness; human nature is like the grass that shoots forth but soon withers and dies (Ps 90:5-6; 103:15-16; Is 40:6-8). Waldemar Janzen sums up his work with these images and shows their relevance to our understanding of the healing ministry:

> Who is the human creature, according to God's design? We have considered three key terms so far: (*adam*) "of the earth"; (*nephesh*) "needy person"; and (*basar*) "vulnerable person." That is a humble picture. The Bible teaches us to understand human beings by understanding their lowliness, their need, and their weakness. That is not the whole story, but it is a good starting base.[5]

---

[4]Willard M. Swartley, *Israel's Faith Traditions and the Synoptic Gospels: Story Shaping Story* (Peabody, Mass.: Hendrickson, 1994), pp. 9-10.
[5]Waldemar Janzen, "Human Wholeness in Biblical Perspective," in *Still in the Image: Essays in*

The Psalms often emphasize this dimension of human life, our frailty and finitude (e.g., Ps 39; 90; 103:14-16). The psalmist cries to God, "how fleeting my life is" and then finally says that he is only a "passing guest, an alien, like all my forebears" (Ps 39:4, 12).

Yet, bleakness about the human condition is not the final word. We are made in the divine image, called to reflect God in this world. In the Genesis story we have been given the capacity for dominion over all the earth. With God, we can *co*create, but God alone is Creator. We can think, speak, remember and plan for the future. We can reflect critically on our own thinking, correct our mistakes, and seek to "construct" our universe in ways more amenable to our needs and desires, responding to the desired comfort of our bodies, minds and spirits. We can experiment, build, travel and procreate, so that our children can carry on the good things we started. As the psalmist puts it, we are "little lower than God" (variant reading, angels) (Ps 8:5). With humanity's fall (Gen 3), however, the image of God in humans is flawed. But it is restored in Christ (Eph 4:20-24). As frail and finite humans, in Christ we become partners with God's creative power.

In view of this need to recognize both our mortality and the human potential of our God image, we must humbly own our mortality and open ourselves to God's work in and through us. For sickness and healing this means affirming God's healing and sustaining power, confessing our frailty and rejoicing in the gift of health. As Mary, my wife, put it after recovering from a serious illness from which she almost died, "Healing is a gift, a gift of grace. That's all there is to say." We own our mortality and humbly affirm God's power to heal and to sustain us in both living and dying. So my prayer:

> God, you are our Creator and we are creatures, human and mortal. We accept the reality of our own dying. We confess that life is a gift from you, a gift of grace. When we are sick and ill, in body or mind or spirit, we look to you for healing. And even when we die, we also claim eternal life through the saving power of Jesus Christ's triumph over death on our behalf.

In January 1993 I participated in a memorial service for Steven Gehman, a thirty-four-year-old seminary graduate who died from an intestinal infection incurred during a second round of chemotherapy. As Steve con-

Biblical Theology and Anthropology (Newton, Kans.: Faith and Life Press, 1982), pp. 62-63.

templated his possible death a few days after he learned he had leukemia, he wrote in his journal:

> Life or death—both are adventures. I can face death because I want God's Kingdom to come more than anything else in the world. And I know that the coming of God's Kingdom will not be delayed if I should die soon.

What a marvelous testimony. Through affirming Christian faith in the face of his death we were brought nearer to God's heart. His life and death served a larger cause.

GOD AS HEALER

One of the means God revealed Yahweh's healing power for the redeemed community through was the name "Yahweh-heals" (*rapha*; Ex 15:26). In various verbal and nominal forms, *rapha* occurs eighty-six times in the Hebrew Scripture.[6] Gaiser notes that the Hebrew here (*rōpê'ekā*) can be translated "I am the LORD, your healer" (RSV); "I am the LORD who heals you" (NRSV); or Luther's translation, "I am the LORD, your physician" (Ich bin der Herr, dein Arzt).[7] This divine self-revelation comes at the end of Israel's early song celebrating release from bondage. The memorable Moses and Miriam music festival celebrates God's sustaining life for them from the waters of death and from the life of slavery. At the end of this chapter, it reads, "If you will listen carefully to the voice of the LORD your God, and do what is right in his sight, and give heed to his commandments and keep all his statues, I will not bring upon you any of the diseases that I brought upon the Egyptians; for I am the LORD who heals you" (*Yahweh-rapha*). And then "they came to Elim, where there were twelve springs of water and seventy palm trees; and they camped there by the water" (see also Num 33:9). Quite a shalom-healthful environment!

Here (as in chap. 3, with Jesus' proclaiming the kingdom of God) salvation and healing are closely linked,[8] as are shalom and healing (see chap. 11). We need to emphasize these connections in our theology and teaching of Scripture: God gives health and is our healer. The God of Israel's Scripture

---

[6]Brown, *Israel's Divine Healer*, p. 25. Brown has a detailed discussion of the range of uses, pp. 25-35.
[7]Frederick Gaiser, *Healing in the Bible: Theological Insights for Christian Ministry* (Grand Rapids: Baker Academic, 2010), p. 21 n. 1.
[8]See note 1 in chap. 3.

is healer with a preventive health care policy, that is, the covenant provisions God set forth for Israel's life. These covenant provisions shape community life, setting forth guidelines for moral behavior and boundaries of conduct to enhance health and wholeness. Covenant shapes the cultic and moral life of the people. The crucial text is Exodus 19–20. In the New Testament we might similarly regard the Lord's Supper covenant, together with the Sermon on the Mount, as central. In both Testaments the covenant community emerges from God's prior act of salvation, liberation of the people from bondage. People are freed to become a new people, to serve and worship the Lord and to relate to each other in life-affirming and community-building ways. Each of the Ten Commandments contributes to the health of the community. Breaking one of them jeopardizes the community's health and welfare. The same is true of Jesus' teaching in the Sermon on the Mount.

The Ten Commandments were given for the community's health. Violating those boundaries generates much psychic pain and causes illness. One of the findings of the World Council of Churches' Christian Medical Commission's study of health care needs says, "in the industrialized nations of the world where modernization has introduced addicting drugs, new diets, and disdain for manual labor, as much as 80 percent of illness is due to self-inflicted destructive life-styles."[9] This datum is linked to environmental threats of nuclear wastes and pollution as well as to personal lifestyle choices.

Two major areas of revolt against the plan God set for humans lie in the areas of sexual lust and economic greed, which often lead to violence (see daily newspaper headlines). Each of the last six commandments is violated frequently in our society as a result of these two forces at work in our Western post-Christian society. While we might name the wealthy newsmakers who have engaged in immoral practices of one kind or another (at least two in 2011), this misses the point. Rather, Western culture is fueled by sex-attracting advertisements and economic profit-making promises. Economic greed has corrupted government big time in recent years, fomented wars and allowed policies that cause environmental pollution, which in part may cause cancer and other illnesses. At the same time, poverty has grown almost exponentially in the last quarter century. In an

---

[9]Karin Granberg-Michaelson, *Healing Community* (Geneva: WCC Publications, 1991), p. 8.

analysis of U.S. income and gains (and losses) for population groupings into five strata (highest income to lowest), the bottom fifth averaged a 122 percent gain between 1947 and 1979, but a loss of 4 percent from 1980-2009. While all five strata had a percentage decline in the last time span only the lowest had a loss. The highest fifth had the largest percent increase in the latter period: 55 percent, compared to the next strata: 25 percent, 15 percent, 7 percent, -4 percent.[10] In hard economic times (e.g., the slight recession in 1982 and the acute one in 2008-2009) the rich become richer and the poor become poorer. Another exposure of America's greed and sexual lust is evident in the crimes reported in our daily local newspapers or newscasts. Almost always these violate one of the last six of the Ten Commandments and are linked to sexual lust or greed.

The church today has a major evangelistic task: to bring itself and our world to call out to Jesus Christ to liberate us from these enslaving, addictive, even demonic powers over and within us. We must take biblical moral teaching seriously, obeying it for the sake of the community's health. We must recognize the devastating effects of our moral choices: smoking, alcoholic consumption, drug use, polluting the environment, sexual abuse, immoral sexual behaviors, pornography and abusive uses of power in the workplace and home.

The matter of personal religious allegiance also has bearing on health issues. The Lord God's promise of health to the newly redeemed Israelite people in Exodus 15:26 holds only if Israel remains faithful in covenant loyalty to this God. The context of this promise is the Lord's sending plagues against the Egyptians. Salvation from bondage and promised health are inherently related. Frederick Gaiser's treatment of this text is insightful. He connects verse 26 with verse 23, in which the bitter waters are "healed" so the newly freed Israelites can drink them.[11] The "bitterness" is symbolic of Israel's rebellion, occurring frequently in Exodus and Numbers. The Lord's promise to protect from disease and heal is thus conditional. If Israel "will (1) listen carefully to the voice of God, (2) do what is right in God's sight, and (3) give heed to God's commandments and keep all his statutes, God will not bring on them any of the diseases

---

[10]*Christian Century*, October 4, 2011, p. 9; source, *New York Times*, September 4. In discussing poverty worldwide, Richard Stearns, president of World Vision, touches lightly on poverty in America, but does say "Poverty in America is just as real as in Africa" (*The Hole in Our Gospel* [Nashville: Thomas Nelson, 2009], p. 118). Poverty affects health, limiting health care access.

[11]Gaiser, *Healing in the Bible*, p. 22.

that were brought upon the Egyptians."[12] If on the other hand, they make idols to worship the gods of the nations, then the diseases of these peoples, as well as God's judgments, will come upon them too (Ex 32 makes the point; see v. 35). The "I AM" Lord alone is to be obeyed and worshiped. The Lord both wounds and heals (Deut 32:39; cf. Is 45:7).

Here is a dramatic correlation between religion and health. But we know not all so-called Christian religion produces good health, so we must be careful how we use this biblical teaching. It is not a magical formula. Israel's history shows both God's faithfulness to heal (e.g., Hezekiah) as well as God's punishment through plagues of disease or natural destruction (e.g., Lev 26:14-33; Num 16:1-35).

In this day of religious pluralism we must think anew about God loyalty, its offer of salvation that makes us whole and the protective power afforded by that salvation. We know the consequences on health care of misplaced religious loyalty. Much ill health has been generated in the last half-century by religious and moral choices against God. (Think only of all the disabled on both sides of the many wars fought.) Nor have we comprehended fully the cause and effect relationship between war making and illness (especially from the use of Agent Orange and depleted uranium). Add to this the sexual practices that contribute to HIV/AIDS. We have not adequately honored the biblical instruction for the moral life that enhances the health of the community.

Our understanding of health must include God's intended way for human living. For this reason, shalom and health are interrelated. God wills shalom for the people of the covenant, and relationship to God in the covenant contributes to that shalom. Malachi, lamenting the unfaithfulness of the covenant people, reminds the people with prophetic passion that they have forsaken God's covenant of *life* and *shalom* (Mal 2:1-10; cf. Ezek 37:24-26).

A text in Proverbs also speaks poetically and powerfully:

> Let your heart hold fast my words;
> keep my commandments and live. . . .
> For they are life to those who find them,
> and healing to all their flesh (Prov 4:4, 22).

---

[12]Ibid., p. 23.

This voice of wisdom (*sophia*) continues in Proverbs 8, calling us to "the fear of the LORD" and to hate evil: perverted speech, pride and arrogance, and trusting in riches. Faithful relation to God is foundational for faith communities to mediate God's healing.

In this call to follow God's way for the sake of our corporate health I do not accept a simplistic formula that is expressed at times in Scripture that all sickness is caused by sin, in a one to one cause-and-effect relationship. That too is wrong (Job; Jn 9:1-3). However, we have erred too much on the side of not teaching clearly enough that immoral conduct and illness are interconnected. Scientific evidence supports the point, but the Old Testament prophets saw it as the result of disobedience to God's covenant law (Hos 4:1-3 and Mic 6:1-8 are clear on this). Both texts also link environmental catastrophe to the people's sins and idolatries. The Old Testament prophets didn't have scientific evidence, but they knew that morality and spirituality are related to the well-being of the person, community and cosmos. The church has an important teaching ministry to instruct about behaviors and habits that promote the health and healing of God's people.

SICKNESS AND HEALING IN THE PSALMS

Many psalms are lament psalms. James Waltner's count is sixty-one, more than one-third of the 150 psalms. Of these he lists forty-five as individual laments and sixteen as communal laments.[13] Lament psalms may also be described as "complaint psalms" since a disparity between the sufferer's condition and God's graciousness and power prompts the psalmist's cry for God to hear and act. Within this genre of lament/complaint are the healing psalms that voice the sufferer in some condition of sickness. Since in some texts illness was understood to be caused by malevolent spiritual powers, and "the enemy" is presented in generalized terms, deliverance and healing psalms overlap. I have listed in table 2.1 both healing and deliverance psalms, in two correlated columns. Many of these psalms contain elements of both healing from illness and deliverance from evil.

---

[13]James H. Waltner, *Psalms*, Believers Church Bible Commentary (Scottdale, Penn.: Herald Press, 2006), p. 787. See also his genre discussion, pp. 762-67 and his type identification of each psalm, pp. 789-91. He does not include healing as a type. They fall into his "individual laments."

These two groups together add up to about thirty, which means other lament psalms focus on other topics, loss of land and nation (Ps 44; 74; 79; 80; 83; 137) or other types of loss (e.g., 55, the loss of a companion who "violated a covenant with me," in vv. 20-21).

The lament/complaint psalms often comment negatively against pagan beliefs, practices or gods (such as Ps 82, accusing king "gods" of not ruling justly). In many of these psalms the psalmist cries out for deliverance from the enemy, portrayed as personal oppression (Ps 3; 5; 12; 18; 68; 118:5-18; etc). Friday Mbon, in his study of complaint psalms, notes that the enemies are not usually identified; they transcend the original historical situation and often refer to the godless or the wicked. He cites Sigmund Mowinckel who suggests that these are "'supernatural beings, demons, or evil spirits,' which he prefers to classify under the general term 'sorcery' (*awen*), and which he suggests, may have been responsible for the psalmists' physical condition in some 'psalms of illness.'"[14]

Steven Croft identifies Psalms 28, 38 and 116 as "prayers in sickness" within the royal psalms; they are prayers by or on behalf of the king.[15] He recognizes that Psalms 6, 13 and 54 have been regarded as prayers for healing from sickness, but he sees in them also a broader focus, praying for deliverance from a variety of dangers. He regards Psalms 30, 41 and 88 as personal cries for healing and notes that both Psalms 30 and 116 are prayers of thanksgiving for healing.[16] For psalms of healing Oepke mentions Psalms 6; 16:10; 32:3-11; 51:7-8.; 103:3; 107:17-43; 147:3.[17] My list includes also Psalms 35 (especially vv. 13-18), 39 and 102.

Psalms 10; 28; 31; 54–57; 126 and 130 have related themes. In many of these psalms the sufferer speaks of God's wrath because of human sin. Sin and guilt are named in some psalms (Ps 6; 38; 41). These psalms and others "bear witness" to the restorative power of confession, producing freedom and renewal within one plagued by guilt as that person is embraced in divine forgiveness.[18]

---

[14]Friday Mbon, "Deliverance in the Complaint Psalms: Religious Claim or Religious Experience," *Studies in Biblical Theology* 12 (1982): 9.

[15]Steven J. L. Croft, *The Identity of the Individual in the Psalms* (Sheffield, UK: JSOT, 1987), pp. 128-29.

[16]Ibid., pp. 137-40.

[17]A. Oepke, "ἰάομαι," in *Theological Dictionary of the New Testament,* ed. Gerhard Kittel and Gerhard Friedrich (Grand Rapids: Eerdmans, 1965), 3:202.

[18]On Ps 38 see Gaiser, *Healing in the Bible,* pp. 78-85; for Ps 6, pp. 8-20.

Table 2.1. Psalms of Healing

Healing Psalms	Deliverance Psalms
6	3
13	5
16:9-11	12
	18
25:16-18	25:20-21
30	27
32:3f.	
35	
38	
39	
40	40
41	
51	59
	68
88	91
102	
103:3	
107:17ff.	
116	118
147:3	

Isaiah 38:10-20, Hezekiah's prayer for healing, fits also the healing psalm type. The Lord heard and answered his prayer, healed him and added fifteen years to his life.[19]

In healing psalms illness is viewed as an interruption of God's shalom order of creation at the personal level. One writer describes these psalms from this perspective:

> The contents of these Psalms reveal a discrepancy between the *shalom* of the order of creation and the well-being of the individual within that order, which was often described as suffering illness, economic distress, or the animosity of personal enemies. It was the aim of the lament to restore the petitioner to a condition of wholeness in relation to the cosmic order.[20]

---

[19]Hezekiah's response contrasts to Asa's. Asa not only appealed to physicians not associated with Israel's God, but he did not call on the Lord to heal (2 Chron 16:7-10; ibid., p. 30). Like Hezekiah, in 1999 I asked God for fifteen years, the Lord willing, for God may be gracious.

[20]Jonathan Paige Sisson, "Jeremiah and the Jerusalem Conception of Peace," *Journal of Biblical Literature* 105 (1986): 432; see notes 8-11, 17-20 for the meaning and uses of shalom in Old Testament literature.

The prevailing view of the Psalms is that sickness is loss of shalom. Illness is understood as a result of many factors (see fig. 2.1), but basically it means loss of shalom. Communal relationships, both at work and in family, play into the many factors causing illness and assisting wellness. Healing is restoring shalom, again with the aid of many factors, including new supportive relationships (see fig. 2.2). These Venn diagrams describe the surrounding Gestalt situations of both illness and wellness in Old Testament understanding. These factors causatively play into sickness and wellness, from an Old Testament Hebrew point of view. Psalm 38:3 voices some of these emphases:

> There is no soundness in my flesh
>   because of your indignation;
> there is no health [shalom] in my bones
>   because of my sin.

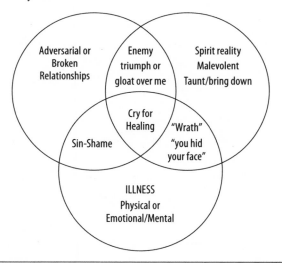

Figure 2.1. No shalom

At the heart of illness is the cry to God for help, such as in Psalm 5:1-2 or Psalm 30:2, 10: "O LORD my God, I cried to you for help" and "Hear, O LORD, and be gracious to me! / O LORD, be my helper!" At the heart of healing is restored shalom (fig. 2.2), with bursts of "Praise and Thanksgiving" to God as healer, such as Psalm 13:5-6, "I trusted in your steadfast love; my heart shall rejoice in your salvation. I will sing to the Lord, because he has dealt bountifully with me."

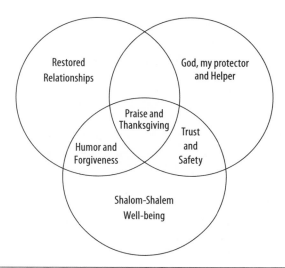

Figure 2.2. Shalom

In his dissertation on the relation of *shalom* to health and healing, Savage identifies numerous psalm texts that speak of some form of this relation: Psalms 6:2; 30:2; 41:4; 60:2; 107:20; and 147:2, which he examines in detail.[21] In these texts the Hebrew *rapha* (to heal) occurs. In the semantic field of *shalom* belong steadfast love (*hesed*), righteousness, justice, obedience, strength, fertility and longevity.[22] Savage correlates healing with these motifs in these psalms. In sum,

> Reclamation of *shalom* is the main objective sought for by the psalmist(s), and healing from Yahweh's *hesed* and grace is the operative force that restores the fractured relationships(s) between Yahweh and His people. The fracturing of personal or communal relationships with Yahweh is portrayed by characteristics of physical, mental, spiritual, social or national turmoil. The cry for healing is predominantly a cry against evil, hoping for the forgiveness of sin or the subduing of enemies that caused the fracturing of *shalom*. Yahweh's *rapha* results in a condition of *shalom*, whereby the petitioner of Yahweh's mercy is restored to a harmonious *shalom*/health relationship with God.[23]

---

[21]Joseph M. Savage, "Shalom and Its Relationship to Health/Healing in the Hebrew Scriptures: A Contextual and Semantic Study of the Books of Psalms and Jeremiah" (Ph.D. diss., Florida State University, 2001), pp. 27-43.

[22]Wilkinson, *Bible and Healing*, p. 63.

[23]Savage, "Shalom," p. 45. Savage also identifies and discusses aspects of shalom (safety) and

Psalm 30 traverses three stages of experience: original shalom (v.6), the disorientation of sickness and cry for help and healing (vv. 2, 8-10), and restoration to "new life" in which mourning is turned into dancing, so "that my soul may praise you and not be silent" (vv. 3, 11-12).[24]

> O LORD my God, I cried to you for help,
>> and *you have healed me.*
> O LORD, you brought up my soul from Sheol,
>> restored me to life from among those gone down to the Pit.
> Sing praises to the LORD, O you his faithful ones,
>> and give thanks to his holy name.
> For his anger is but for a moment;
>> his favor is for a lifetime.
> Weeping may linger for the night,
>> but joy comes with the morning.
> As for me, I said in my prosperity,
>> "I shall never be moved."
> By your favor, O LORD,
>> you had established me as a strong mountain;
> you hid your face;
>> I was dismayed.
> To you, O LORD, I cried,
>> and to the LORD I made supplication:
> "What profit is there in my death,
>> if I go down to the Pit?
> Will the dust praise you?
>> Will it tell of your faithfulness?
> Hear, O LORD, and be gracious to me!
>> O LORD, be my helper!"
> You have turned my mourning into dancing;
>> you have taken off my sackcloth
> and clothed me with joy,
>> *so that my soul may praise you and not be silent.*
> *O LORD my God, I will give thanks to you forever.*
>> (Ps 30:2-12, emphasis added)

This psalm became my biblical mantra during my near-fatal heart attack

---

healing in Ps 4:8; 28:3; 29:11; 34:14; 35:20; 37:11; 55:18; 72:3, 7; 85:8 (cf. Is 32:17); 119:165; 120:6-7; 125:5; 128:6; 147:14 (ibid., pp. 98-102).

[24]Walter Brueggemann, *The Message of the Psalms* (Minneapolis: Augsburg, 1984), pp. 126-27.

(see introduction). The italicized portions nurtured my spirit and aided my will to live and the long, gradual recovery. In this psalm the predominant reason for praising God for healing is that the healed person is free to praise and thank God in an unhindered way. We may know from personal experience that when we are sick or incapacitated, it may be more difficult to praise God. The psalmist felt this and thus ends the psalm: "You have turned my mourning into dancing; / you have taken off my sackcloth / and clothed me with joy, / *so that my soul may praise you and not be silent.* / O Lord my God, I will give thanks to you forever" (emphasis added).[25] Freedom to again praise God contrasts to the dread of death (v. 9), "What profit is there in my death, / if I go down to the Pit? / Will the dust praise you? / Will it tell of your faithfulness?"

Songwriter James Seddon (1973), with stanza 4 added later by Calvin Seerveld (1982), put Psalm 30 into worship mode:

I worship you, O Lord for you have raised me up;
    I cried to you for help, and you restored my life.
You brought me back from death and saved me from the grave

Sing praises to the Lord, all those who know his name;
    for while his wrath is brief, his favour knows no end.
Though tears may flow at night, the morning brings new joy.

I said, "I am so strong, I never shall be moved!";
    but you, Lord, shook my life—my heart was in distress.
I cried for you to help and pleaded for your grace.

"What good am I when dead, while lying in the grave?
    Can dust recount your love, the grave proclaim your praise?
O hear me, gracious Lord, in mercy be my aid!"

My mourning you have turned to dancing and to joy;
    my sadness you dispelled as gladness filled my soul.
And so I'll sing your praise, my God, through all my days![26]

---

[25] Lori Vincent, having had sixteen cancer surgeries over the past twelve years, beating all odds for survival, gave a powerful sermon at Belmont Mennonite Church in fall 2011, marked energetically with praise of God, lauding and thanking the Lord's graciousness, and crediting also the expertise and caring of numerous medical personnel. See *Fighting Disease, Not Death: Finding a Way Through Lifelong Struggle*, by Lori L. Vincent and Mark L. Vincent (Indianapolis: Dog Ear, 2011).

[26] James E. Seddon, "I Worship You, O Lord" (1973). As I was working on this chapter in 2008, I was introduced to this moving text and tune by Christian worship professor John Witvliet

Seerveld's addition to Seddon's text is important, for it voices this biblical, certainly Old Testament, fear that death silences praise of God. The hymn text might have further emphasized this point by including "and not be silent" of verse 12. The silencing of praise to God is the psalmist's dread. But the psalmist's healing releases his voice to sing God's praise all his remaining days! Even in Psalm 22, with its "God-forsakenness" (see vv. 1-21; v. 1 was quoted by Jesus on the cross [Mk 15:34]), is punctuated by verse 3, "Yet you are holy, / enthroned on the praises of Israel." The long dour lament turns into praise and testimony in verses 22-31.

Another strand of biblical teaching stresses that even in sickness and suffering we can and do trust and praise God. Marva Dawn's life, fraught with physical infirmity, and her writings, testify to the truth that infirmities need not hinder praise of God. She writes on this point:

> I could find no texts that say anything about any incapacity to serve God when our infirmities encumber us. In several passages such as . . . [Ps 6:4-5, her epigraph for the chapter] (see also Ps. 30:9; 88:10-12; 115:7; Eccles. 9:10; Isa. 38:18) the poet asks to be delivered from death and the grave because no one can praise the Lord there.[27]

We cannot view sickness and suffering only negatively. On the one hand, sickness and suffering appear to fight against God, as legacy from the evil one in humanity's fall, but Scripture also points to a positive response to God amid suffering. At the deepest level, through trusting in God, suffering is a means of endearment to the heart of God, for God hears the cry of the sufferer.[28]

Job's witness plumbs the depths of the sufferer's agony and quest for meaning in suffering. We learn from Job that humans cannot presume to know the ways of God. In the midst of suffering God is still there; and *the righteous sufferer is a friend of God*. Jesus as sufferer is God's answer to us; in Jesus God suffers with us. He bears our infirmities, both with us and for us. In suffering we cry to God to help and to heal and to carry us. Amid suffering, we can also praise God—perhaps even more purely, as did the psalmist in

---

(Calvin College and Seminary), who was presenting a lecture at Anabaptist Mennonite Biblical Seminary. Used with permission from © Hope Publishing Co. for stanzas 1, 2, 3 and 5 and from Calvin Seerveld for stanza 4.

[27] Marva Dawn, *Being Well When We're Ill: Wholeness and Hope in Spite of Infirmity* (Minneapolis: Augsburg, 2008), p. 130. See her prayer on p. 140.

[28] C. S. Lewis, *The Problem of Pain* (New York: Macmillan, 1963).

Psalm 22:3-4, 22-31. Nevertheless, healing evokes outbursts of praise to God.

At least a dozen psalms illumine the Hebrew view of sickness and healing as both the disruption and restoration of shalom. In many of these psalms the sufferer cries out for help and healing: "O Lord my God, I cried to you for help, / and you have healed me" (Ps 30:2). In Psalm 6 we see the tears of the sick person (cf. Ps 56:8). Illness is viewed as death encroaching (Ps 30:3); the psalmist's worst terror is not being able to praise God. Bernhard Anderson observes, "The view of life and death presupposed in the psalms is quite different from modern biological conceptions . . . [i.e.,] the heart stops beating and consciousness goes out like a light." According to the Israelite view, death brings about "a decrease in the vitality of the individual." Death's power is felt in

> the midst of life to the degree that one experiences any weakening of personal vitality through illness, handicap, imprisonment, attack from enemies, or advancing old age. Any threat to a person's welfare (Hebrew *shalom*, peace, well-being), that is, one's freedom to be and to participate in the covenant community, is understood as an invasion of the empire of death into the historical arena.[29]

For the psalmists the tragedy of death is that it transposes people into another, nonhistorical realm where they can no longer praise God.

Psalms 90 and 103 acknowledge that human life is frail and brief. Psalm 90 contrasts God's eternality to the fleeting span of human life: like grass that flourishes in the morning, and "in the evening it fades and withers" (Ps 90:6). While the normal life span is seventy years, yet even with eighty, life is filled with "trouble; they are soon gone, and we fly away" (Ps 90:10). Psalm 103 memorably lauds God's compassion and forgiveness, but also memorably expresses life's fragility:

> [God] knows how we were made;
> he remembers that we are dust.
> As for mortals, their days are like grass;
> they flourish like a flower of the field;
> for the wind passes over it, and it is gone,
> and its place knows it no more. (Ps 103:14-16)

---

[29]Bernhard W. Anderson, *Out of the Depths* (Philadelphia: Westminster Press, 1983), pp. 122, 127.

While the latter may fit some of the psalm depictions of sickness, the language is stylized and void of detail, as Anderson notes, and thus readily expresses the cries of sufferers through the ages.[30] Is personal sin, iniquity or transgression considered cause for illness in the Psalms? The answer depends on how widely one casts the net in selecting psalms of sickness. If we include Psalms 32 and 51, as Oepke does, then these together with Psalms 39 (vv. 8, 11) and 41 (v. 4, "heal me, for I have sinned against you") make an explicit link between sickness and sin. The poetic parallel between sins and diseases in Psalm 103:3 is not a causal connection, in my judgment. If we also include the psalms that reflect more generalized distress, including the deliverance psalms[31] (3, 5, 12, 18, 59, 68, 91, 118) the number is much greater in which some person or thing is considered a causal agent. Hence the self-vindication and plea to God consist of stating one's faithfulness to God against the intent of the enemy (Ps 6:8, 10; 13:2-4; 41:4-12).[32]

Psalm 103, a jubilant song of thanksgiving for healing, shows that the experience of illness and recovery generates deepened appreciation for God's mighty works of salvation and steadfast love—true of my experience, grasping on to Psalm 30:11-12. The sufferer is restored to where he or she can again praise God, function freely in the community and thus reclaim shalom. Psalm 23 is usually not identified as a healing psalm. It does not topically fit the mold but it is a psalm that brings comfort and healing balm. Perhaps it should be included in the healing psalm list. Hear and pray it, reciting it by heart!

A *third* powerful healing perspective from Old Testament thought is

---

[30]Ibid., pp. 85-86. Brown lists eleven themes present in these Psalms (*Israel's Divine Healer*, pp. 122-23), which my discussion also mentions.

[31]Of the deliverance psalms, Psalm 91 was used in early Judaism as a psalm for exorcism. Unfortunately, our translations do not show the exorcist emphasis as clearly as they might. Two words in verse 6 refer to nighttime and daytime demons: *opel*, translated "pestilence" in NRSV and *qetev*, translated "destruction" in NRSV. It is indeed ironic that the devil used this psalm to tempt Jesus (in Mt 4 and Lk 4) into thinking that God would send angels to bear him up if he would jump off the temple at the devil's instigation. I suppose the devil had heard this psalm frequently in exorcism and now misuses it. It is a psalm against him, not for him. And Jesus rightly responds, "Do not put the Lord your God to the test," quoting from Deuteronomy 6:16. Even scriptural truth in the devil's mouth is deception and presumption.

[32]If Psalm 25 is included as a psalm of sickness, based on vv. 16-18, then it cites both personal sins (vv. 7, 18) and foes (vv. 2, 19) as causative. Psalm 88 mentions neither; in it mental anguish is most intense.

that God as Divine Warrior is at work to overcome death and its power. Isaiah 25:6-9 is one such passage:

> On this mountain the LORD of hosts will make for all peoples
>> a feast of rich food, a feast of well-aged wines,
>> of rich food filled with marrow, of well-aged wines strained clear.
> And he will destroy on this mountain
>> the shroud that is cast over all peoples,
>> the sheet that is spread over all nations;
> he will swallow up death forever.
>> Then the Lord GOD will wipe away the tears from all faces,
>> and the disgrace of his people he will take away from all the earth,
>> for the LORD has spoken.
> It will be said on that day,
>> Lo, this is our God; we have waited for him, so that he might save us.
>> This is the LORD for whom we have waited;
>> let us be glad and rejoice in his salvation.

The Psalms envision life beyond death.[33] Here are my personal favorites:

> You show me the path of life.
>> In your presence there is fullness of joy;
>> in [at] your right hand are pleasures forevermore. (Ps 16:11)

> As for me, I shall behold your face in righteousness;
>> when I awake I shall be satisfied, beholding your likeness. (Ps 17:15)

> You guide me with your counsel,
>> and afterward you will receive me with honor [into glory]. . . .
> My flesh and my heart may fail,
>> but God is the strength of my heart and my portion forever. (Ps 73:24, 26)

Leonard Greenspoon sees God's cosmic battle against chaos, begun at creation, continuing in divine warfare and culminating in overcoming the power of death itself.[34] Thus Isaiah 25:6-10; 35; Ezekiel 37; and Daniel

---

[33]Mitchell Dahood counters the dominant view that life beyond death is not found in the Old Testament. See his *Psalms*, Anchor Bible (Garden City, N.Y.: Doubleday, 1966), p. xxxvi, where he lists eleven psalm verses that connote hope of life beyond death. These texts include my three favorites Ps 16:11; 17:15; 73:24, 26. In addition, he includes Ps 1:3-6; 5:9; 11:7; 21:6; 27:13; 36:9-10; 37:37-38; 56:13.

[34]Leonard Greenspoon, "The Origin of the Idea of the Resurrection," in *Traditions in Transformation: Turning Points in Biblical Faith*, ed. Baruch Halpern and Jon D. Levenson (Winona Lake, Ind.: Eisenbrauns, 1981), pp. 247-321.

12:1-3 are the endpoints of God's victory within the Old Testament. This is a different angle than the usual interpretation that the doctrine of the resurrection has only slight beginnings in the Old Testament. But this emphasis approaches it from the other side, namely, the victory of God. Jewish scholar Jon Levenson also challenges the older view. He argues that resurrection is deeply embedded in the Hebrew Scripture, especially in the corporate sense of God's covenant promise to Israel.[35] God's promise is victory over death. From a Christian perspective this culminates in Jesus Christ's triumph over death; he is the resurrection and the life (Jn 11:25).

These psalms come "close" when we are ill, physically, emotionally, mentally or spiritually. We join them also to Jesus Christ, as our Savior and healer. Especially in those psalms where illness is interconnected with sin, we come to Jesus Christ to ask forgiveness for our sin, to humbly and truly confess it. In Jesus Christ forgiveness of sins is fully assured, lifting guilt and shame, and freeing us from malevolent powers. God's healing power in Jesus Christ renews our spirits and heals our minds and bodies.

The healing psalms provide a model for our own prayers of healing to God.[36] My older brother Henry, who died January 13, 1988, left behind a rich journal legacy. In his failing health he cried to God for healing. Though not cured of his heart illness, he found healing:

> Lord and Father of all humankind,
>> Creator, sustainer, helper, healer, and savior.
> I come with a burden of great anguish.
>> With deep crying in my soul
> And pain in my body, my heart, and my mind.
>> Lord, that is my health problem
>
> I cried out to You for divine healing.
>> I've tried to submit to You in suffering.

---

[35]Jon D. Levenson, *Resurrection and the Restoration of Israel: The Ultimate Victory of the God of Life* (New Haven, Conn.: Yale University Press, 2006).

[36]This is superbly done by Ann Weems in *Psalms of Lament* (Louisville: Westminster John Knox, 1995). Her laments were prompted by the harsh death of her twenty-one-year-old son. These laments also show that lament is a broader category than healing psalms, evident also in Nicholas Wolterstorff's *Lament for a Son* (Grand Rapids: Eerdmans, 1987), chap. 4, and Rachel Nafziger Hartzler's chapter on lament, occasioned by the sudden death of her husband, *Grief and Sexuality: Life After Losing a Spouse* (Scottdale, Penn.: Herald Press, 2006), pp. 51-76. Lament is the psalm genre for losses, not only loss of health.

I exert all my faith, believing that You are healing.
I have watched my diet, hoping that would help.
I have exercised and walked when I hardly could,
But yet healing seems afar off.

[Two stanzas omitted]

Yet in the stillness of this hour I know You are there.
I know that You are the great Healer.
I know Your divine purposes are in the works.
I hear Your still small Voice whispering love.
I saw You in Vision and experienced You in dreams.
I know Your healing hand is upon me and upon all your children.

[Four stanzas omitted]

I give back my life to You, O Lord, in life or death,
health or sickness, whole or infirmed.
I pledge my remaining days to serve You and
to bring Your life to a few more persons who are crying.
And most of all, I just want to worship You
in the beauty of Your holiness on earth and in heaven. Amen.[37]

EXCURSUS

Numerous types of healing permeate our society, alongside the worldviews of Judeo-Christian faith and scientific medical resources. Some scholars hold, however, that the Judeo-Christian worldview enabled scientific healing to develop, since it desacralized nature, allowing for empirical study (*scientia:* knowing through observation and experiment). Outside this Western worldview is the larger global healing reality. As Stephen Parsons puts it in *The Challenge of Christian Healing,* "we should bear in mind that 'healers' operating outside a Christian framework are probably more numerous than those who use a Christian understanding."[38]

Parsons, like Morton Kelsey, too readily moves from healing generally to Christian healing in stories they cite. At the root of this issue is whether natural abilities to discern and heal (i.e., those born with these special powers) are the same as what Paul calls "gifts of healing" from the Holy

---

[37]Henry Swartley, "Midnight Prayer," in *Living on the Fault-Line: Journals and Portrait of Church Planter Pastor*, ed. Willard Swartley (Nappanee, Ind.: Evangel Press, 1992), pp. 24-25.
[38]Stephen Parsons, *The Challenge of Christian Healing* (London: SPCK, 1986), p. viii.

Spirit. Some Christians regard these "natural" abilities (which include clairvoyant powers and water dowsing, for example) as negative spirit power (i.e., demonic), as they are passed from generation to generation. Discernment is needed in this crucial area.

I find Parsons's definition of healing helpful:

> By "healing" we mean a capacity in an individual or group to change for the good the course of a disease in another, whether physical or psychological in nature. This capacity to heal is variously regarded as a psychic or spiritual gift, and appears to involve the tapping of energies which so far are beyond the realm of conventional science to explain. Healing may also sometimes be understood as the calling forth of an individual's own self-healing powers by some as yet little-understood psychic communication between healer and patient.[39]

While Christian and non-Christian healers both tap into a power or energy beyond human understanding, perceptions differ regarding the source of the healing energy: non-Christians may call it the energy of the universe (as in new age healing) whereas Christians see it as God's, Christ's and the Holy Spirit's power mediated through believers.

A theology and practice of Christian healing does not begin with answers to the many questions about the mechanics of what makes it work, but with the obedient response to Christ to heal the sick as part of proclaiming the gospel.[40] Further, Christian healing results in a renewed relationship to Christ, the Holy Spirit and God, whereas new age healing often speaks of cosmic force or energy. Christians therefore are rightly suspicious of the source of healing power outside the explicitly Christian framework. Some may be counterfeit healings by evil power (witness Simon the magician in Acts 8:9-24); when these healings are confronted with Christ as healer they will be undone and true healing in the name of Jesus occurs.[41]

These are the context issues that the church increasingly faces in our Western society. We must take more seriously both the task of discernment

---

[39]Ibid., p. vii.

[40]Ibid., p. viii.

[41]I have witnessed this in regard to the Amish magical practices of powwow. This is practiced less and less among the Amish, as they welcome Jesus Christ as healer and receive medical care.

and the church's belief in healing in other than the scientific health care mode. And this, of course, raises another contextual issue. How is scientific health care or medical healing related to Christian healing? In the same way, I propose, that scientific study of the Bible is related to Scripture being the Word of God for us. In both cases the good scientific practitioner recognizes that the healing process or event of God addressing us is a divine action, not fully in our grasp or know-how. Scientific health care sets the stage for God's healing to occur, through the marvelous process God put within our bodies. Scripture scholars similarly prepare the way: giving historical and cultural background or structural and definitional information that enable the Word to bridge the gap between the biblical text and our ministries, including healing (Gaiser's *Healing in the Bible* is a fine contribution to this "bridging of the gap").

Christians, therefore, can embrace scientific health care contributions and Christian healing as compatible and mutually conducive to wellness. Certainly we both pray for healing and seek medical services. Hard questions, however, must be asked regarding: the limits of scientific effort vis à vis trust in God to heal or accept death; whether non-Western types of medical practices are scientific in ways Western science cannot comprehend or whether they are enabled by energy that taps into the dark powers (on "alternative" healing interventions, note the Bill Moyers series "Healing and the Mind"[42] or the experience of T. R. Reid seeking healing for his lame shoulder in a half-dozen cultures with differing types of medical care and healing). The relation between healing prayer and deliverance prayer is also important. How do we discern when to command evil powers to leave and go to Jesus for judgment so that a person is free to become well?

These questions are not easy to answer in abstraction, and perhaps even harder in specific real-life situations. Sensitive spiritual discernment and humble prayer to God guide one's response to varied situations. But this we say confidently: Jesus' healing and deliverance ministries are part of our gospel calling. The work of health care professionals is part of God's mission in the world (chap. 8). Church ministries need to work with doctors and nurses, combining healing prayer and scientific health care efforts.

---

[42]The collection of essays titled *Healing and the Mind* is helpful on this topic. See Bill Moyers, *Healing and the Mind*, ed. Betty Sue Flowers, David Grubin and Elizabeth Meryman-Brunner (New York: Doubleday, 1995), as well as more recent TV programs by Moyers.

3

❖

Healing in the New Testament
and the Church's Practice

*You know the message he [God] sent to the people of Israel, preaching
peace by Jesus Christ . . . [and] he went about doing good and healing all
who were oppressed by the devil, for God was with him.*

Acts 10:36, 38

Luke's summary of Jesus' ministry stuns. The Gospels are laced with healing stories. In John 9 Jesus heals a man born blind. Three issues and insights emerge for our contemporary thinking about healing.

He describes Jesus as a peace preacher and healer. First, the story breaks any formulaic connection between illness and sin in a one-to-one relationship. While there is a connection between the lifestyles of people and the health of a community, any explicit direct connection to sin for a given person must be refused. Rather than imputing blame to someone for his or her illness, the point is rather that the whole community suffers from wrong choices and priorities. Sickness is ultimately rooted in the fallen state of humanity; all creation is implicated as well.

Second, healing is an essential aspect of Jesus' gospel, related to the disclosure of his identity. In this miracle of John 9 faith is not a precondition for the blind man's healing, but Jesus' healing prompts both faith and unbelief, with the latter mounting as the chapter progresses. The religious unbelieving leaders are "the blind" (vv. 40-41); the blind man now *sees*. He is the model believer (vv. 35-38). *Seeing the light* happens when we say yes to what Jesus can do for us, affirming the blind man's christological perception and confession. It is *physical* sight for the blind man; for most of us it is *spiritual*. What faith response does Jesus' deed evoke in us?

Third, here arises an important issue in discernment for Christian ministry. Pastors and church leaders are encountering different types of "healers," some in the Eastern religious traditions. This story suggests that to discern the nature of the healing gift, we should talk about Jesus as Prophet-Savior, Son of Man, and Lord-healer. John 9, together with other New Testament stories, joins healing and Christology.

JESUS: SAVIOR AND HEALER ESSENTIAL
TO HIS KINGDOM AND MISSION

The Gospel writers use a variety of terms to describe Jesus' healing ministry. Most frequent is *therapeuō*, from which our English word *therapy* is derived. Its basic meaning is "to serve," in relation to a deity. But it also means care for someone and *curing* of illness. Second in frequency is *iaomai*, which means to heal or cure. Both terms were also in the medical vocabulary of the Greek world. Sometimes the verb for salvation, *sōzō*, is used to describe physical healing in the New Testament (e.g., Mk 5:34); the person is saved, healed from his or her illness.[1] Still another word, *hygiainō*, designates a healthy or sound state of body, mind and spirit. From it comes our word *hygiene*. To this vocabulary in the Gospels we add also Paul's mention of the charismatic gift of healing (1 Cor 12:9, 28, 30). Here healing is based in *charisma*, a direct gift of God.

In the Gospels healings were an essential part of Jesus' mission. These healings and exorcisms announced the in-breaking of God's reign and certified Jesus' messianic claims. Walter Wink, in *Engaging the Powers*, says,

> Jesus' healings and exorcisms, which play such a major role in his ministry, are not simply patches on a body destined for death regardless; they are manifestations of God's reign now, an inbreaking of eternity into time, a revelation of God's merciful nature, a promise of the restitution of all things

---

[1]Donald Gowan, "Salvation as Healing," *Ex Auditu* 5 (1989): 1-19; James Lapsley, *Salvation and Health: The Interlocking Process of Life* (Philadelphia: Westminster Press, 1972); and Wolfgang Schrage, "Heil und Heilung im Neuen Testament," in *Kreuzestheologie und Ethik im Neuen Testament* (Göttingen: Vandenhoeck & Ruprecht, 2004), pp. 87-105.

in the heart of the loving Author of the universe. . . . God's nonviolent reign
is the overcoming of demonic powers through nonviolent means.[2]

Scholars agree (healing miracles were a significant part of Jesus' ministry. Joel Green counts eighteen healings and four healing summaries in
Mark, nineteen and four in Matthew, twenty and three in Luke. John has
four healing signs, including his climactic one: raising dead Lazarus to
life.[3] Morton Kelsey says nearly "one-fifth of the entire Gospels is devoted
to Jesus' healings and discussions occasioned by them."[4] In comparison,
scant attention is given to moral healing (Matthew, Zacchaeus, the Samaritan woman at the well in Jn 4, the sinful woman in Lk 7:37-50, and
the woman taken in adultery by the Pharisees in Jn 8:3-11). Kelsey counts
forty-one distinct instances (seventy-two with duplications: see table 3.1).
He identifies the method of healing and exorcism: by word only, touch,
preaching or other action. Both Kelsey and Stanger list them separately
and ask readers to reassess their understanding of salvation in light of
Jesus' priority.[5]

A dominant portrait of the historical Jesus is that of healer and exorcist:

> During his lifetime he [Jesus] was known primarily as a healer and exorcist.
> People flocked to him, drawn by his wonder-working reputation, as the
> gospels report again and again: "they brought to him all who were sick or
> possessed with demons. And the whole city was gathered together at the
> door"; as a healer, "His fame spread, and great crowds followed him"; "People
> came to him from every quarter."[6] [Mk 1:32-34; Mt 4:24; Mk 1:45].

When King Herod Antipas heard of Jesus' deeds, he responded in
terror, for he thought John the Baptist, whom he had executed, had risen
from the dead. Even Jesus' opponents did not contest that Jesus did these

---

[2]Walter Wink, *Engaging the Powers: Discernment and Resistance in a World of Domination* (Minneapolis: Fortress Press, 1992), p. 134.

[3]Joel Green, "Healing," in *New Interpreter's Bible Dictionary*, ed. Katharine Doob Sakenfeld
(Nashville: Abingdon, 2007), 2:758.

[4]Morton T. Kelsey, *Healing and Christianity: A Classic Study*, 3rd ed. (Minneapolis: Augsburg,
1995), p. 42.

[5]Ibid., pp. 43-45; Frank Bateman Stanger, *God's Healing Community* (Wilmore, Ky.: Francis
Asbury, 1985), p. 33. Stanger's even longer list is in two sections: "individual" healings (26) and
"multiple healings" (21), some of which are summary statements of healing of "crowds." Only
Kelsey cites the method of healing.

[6]Marcus J. Borg, *Jesus: A New Vision: Spirit, Culture, and a Life of Discipleship* (San Francisco:
Harper & Row, 1987), p. 60.

Table 3.1. Healing Works of Jesus

No.	Healing	Matthew	Mark	Luke	John	Method
1.	Man with unclean spirit		1:23	4:33		Exorcism, word
2.	Peter's mother-in-law	8:14	1:30	4:38		Touch, word; prayer of friends
3.	Multitudes	8:16	1:32	4:40		Touch, word; faith of friends
4.	Many demons		1:39			Preaching, exorcism
5.	A leper	8:2	1:40	5:12		Word, touch; leper's faith and Christ's compassion
6.	Man sick of the palsy	9:2	2:3	5:17		Word; faith of friends
7.	Man's withered hand	12:9	3:1	6:6		Word; obedient faith
8.	Multitudes	12:15	3:10			Exorcism, response to faith
9.	Gerasene demoniac	8:28	5:1	8:26		Word, exorcism
10.	Jairus's daughter	9:18	5:22	8:41		Word, touch; faith of father
11.	Woman with issue of blood	9:20	5:25	8:43		Touching his garment in faith
12.	A few sick folk	13:58	6:5			Touch (hindered by unbelief)
13.	Multitudes	14:34	6:55			Touch of his garment, friend's faith
14.	Syrophoenician's daughter	15:22	7:24			Response to mother's prayer, faith
15.	Deaf and dumb man		7:32			Word, touch; friend's faith
16.	Blind man (gradual healing)		8:22			Word, touch; friends' faith
17.	Child with evil spirit	17:14	9:14	9:38		Word, touch; faith of father
18.	Blind Bartimaeus	20:30	10:46	18:35		Word, touch, compassion, faith
19.	Centurion's servant	8:5		7:2		Response to master's prayer, faith
20.	Two blind men	9:27				Word, touch; men's faith

Table 3.1. Healing Works of Jesus (continued)

No.	Healing	Matthew	Mark	Luke	John	Method
21.	Dumb demoniac	9:32				Exorcism
22.	Blind and dumb demoniac	12:22		11:14		Exorcism
23.	Multitudes	4:23		6:17		Teaching, preaching, healing
24.	Multitudes	9:35				Teaching, preaching, healing
25.	Multitudes	11:4		7:21		Proof of John Bapt. in prison
26.	Multitudes	14:14		9:11	6:2	Compassion, resp. to need
27.	Great multitudes	15:30				Faith of friends
28.	Great multitudes	19:2				
29.	Blind and lame in temple	21:14				
30.	Widow's son			7:11		Word, compassion
31.	Mary Magdalene and others			8:2		Exorcism
32.	Woman bound by Satan			13:10		Word, touch
33.	Man with dropsy			14:1		Touch
34.	Ten lepers			17:11		Word; faith of men
35.	Malchus' ear			22:49		Touch
36.	Multitudes			5:15		
37.	Various persons			13:32		Exorcism, and not stated
38.	Nobleman's son				4:46	Word; father's faith
39.	Impotent man				5:2	Word; man's faith
40.	Man born blind				9:1	Word, touch
41.	Lazarus				11:1	Word

deeds, but sought to discredit him by attributing them to the prince of the demons, Beelzebul (Mt 12:24-28//Mk 3:22-26//Lk 11:15-20). The fourth-century Jewish Talmud continues a similar charge against Jesus, calling him a magician who performed miracles ("practiced sorcery").[7]

This is the Jesus of the Gospels, the archetype of our faith. In Mark 3:13-16 and Mark 6:6-13 Jesus commissions his disciples to participate in his mission. Four points are crucial:

- to be with him (3:14)

- to have authority over unclean spirits

- to proclaim the kingdom of God

- to heal the sick, either laying on of hands or anointing with oil

In Matthew Jesus authorizes the Twelve as follows: "Jesus . . . gave them authority over unclean spirits, to cast them out, and to cure every disease and every sickness" (Mt 10:1). Luke's parallel is: "Jesus . . . gave them power and authority over all demons and to cure diseases, and he sent them out to proclaim the kingdom of God and to heal" (Lk 9:1-2). Luke 10 serves as a prototype of the early church's mission in Acts, in which healing deliverance and proclamation of the kingdom continues.

Bazzana describes the early Christians as both preachers and physicians. Luke 10 and Matthew 10 (and the theoretical Q text that stands behind these) present the physician role of early missionaries. Luke puts healing first and proclamation of the kingdom of God second; Matthew reverses the order.[8]

Of the many points oriented to Jesus' healing ministry, I list seven:

1. In Jesus, a person of great compassion emerges. Jesus had compassion on the sick and the demon-possessed, and desired their freedom and health. Three women freed of demons (Lk 8:1-3, one a wife of Herod's house steward!) later provided financing for the Jesus entourage. Clearly these women, and many others, felt Jesus' compassion. In the Christian tradition compassion is essential for the healing ministry—a compassion that risks self in service to help and heal others (Mt 9:35-38). Without compassion Jesus' ministry would have been nothing more than an ego

---

[7]Babylonian Talmud *Sanhedrin* 43a.

[8]Giovanni Battista Bazzana, "Early Christian Missionaries as Physicians: Healing and Its Cultural Value in the Greco-Roman Context" *Novum Testamentum* 51 (2009): 232-36.

trip. Jesus ministered with complete abandonment of ego; his focus was bringing wholeness to each person he encountered. Without compassion Jesus' words and works would have had no saving significance. In his healings Jesus' person and works of love complement each other.

Compassion is dominant in Jesus' healing ministry; searching for a cause of sickness to impute blame is not. On one occasion Jesus utilizes the common belief that sickness is intertwined with sin; for example, in controversy with the Pharisees over the healing of the paralytic (Mk 2:1-12). But Jesus also separates specific illnesses or catastrophes from *direct causative* sin or evil: in the healing of the man born blind (Jn 9) and in his statement about the Galileans upon whom the tower of Siloam fell (Lk 13:1-5).

2. On several occasions Jesus expresses anger in the face of disease, illness and death. In some manuscripts Jesus gets angry (*orgistheis*) as he encounters the leper in Mark 1:41; most manuscripts though say he had compassion (*splanchnistheis*). But would a scribe change the text from *compassion* to *anger*? The reverse is more likely—with *anger* the original— since the scribal pattern is to change from harder to easier readings, not easier to harder. In John 11:33, when Jesus sees the Jews wailing for Lazarus, Jesus was aggravated (angered or distressed) in spirit, and he cries (v. 35). In Mark 3:5 Jesus gets angry at the Galilean Pharisees' hardness of heart in response to his healing the man with a withered hand. In the first two cases we do not know the cause of Jesus' anger. Perhaps, his anger is stirred by seeing how illness cripples people, obstructs freedom and squeezes out faith and hope. Or perhaps in John 11:33 Lazarus's situation prefigured his own death and resurrection and his weeping is part of his agony to come (cf. Jn 12:27). Whatever the reason, he acts decisively to restore shalom in all these cases. We should not conclude, however, that his mission was solely healing or deliverance. Rather, Jesus' healings testify to Jesus' identity and the dawning of God's reign. They pave the way for the gospel, even today in newly evangelized areas of our world.

3. For these reasons Jesus' healing ministry has an unusual access profile. Most people healed or delivered from demons are not persons with standing in the religious community. The daughter of Jairus, ruler of a synagogue, is an exception (Mk 5:35-42). Even then the *daughter* was healed, not the synagogue ruler. Approximately one-third of those healed

are women. Some persons Jesus healed are ritually defiled. Another third are socially ostracized because they are lepers or demonized. Several are outsiders to the Israelite community: the Syrophoenician woman (Mk 7:24-30), the centurion's servant (Mt 8:5-13) and a royal official's son (Jn 4:46-54).

When we consider the social, economic and religious profile of the people Jesus healed, we learn a basic, important lesson about access. Jesus' healings are not limited to a special group; there are no exclusions. The church is called to continue Jesus' ministry to all people, including the oppressed and marginalized.

4. In numerous cases faith plays a significant role in the healing event. Kelsey identifies *faith* in seventeen of the forty-one cases listed (the word *faith* in the cases of friends or people bringing a person to Jesus usually does not occur, though it may be implied). The woman with a hemorrhage displays exceptional faith (Mk 5:24-34). In Mark's Gospel she alone is commended for her faith. Note the description of the details:

- description of illness: she has a flow of blood for twelve years

- she suffered much from physicians, spent all she had and is no better but only grows worse

- she hears reports of Jesus and presses into the crowd, thinking, "If I but touch his clothes, I will be made well" (v. 28)

- she touches his garment and feels in her body that she is healed of the disease

- Jesus, knowing that power had left him, turns and asks, "Who touched my clothes?" (v. 30)

- Jesus looks around to see who had done it

- The woman comes forth and in "fear and trembling," falls down before him and tells him the whole truth!

- Jesus' commends her faith as basis for her healing

- Jesus' gives a final word of blessing, "Go in peace, and be healed of your disease." (v. 34)

This explicit commendation of the woman's faith and use of the word "peace" (*eirēnē*) is unique to the Markan narrative. When compared to Jesus' word to Jairus, "Do not fear, only believe," it is clear that the woman plays the stronger narrative role, calling the reader to faith in Jesus. Faith is the leitmotif of this entire segment of mighty works (Mk 4:35–6:6). The woman's faith contrasts to the disciples' lack of faith (Mk 4:40) and the unbelief of those in Jesus' hometown (Mk 6:1-6). The contrast puts her faith in bold relief.

5-7. Points five through seven are based on Luke 10:1-20. Luke's Gospel, more clearly than the other three, interrelates three crucial themes: *healing*, proclaiming the peace gospel of the kingdom of God, and the downfall of Satan. This is one whole for Luke, as is clear in Peter's Acts 10:36-38 summary of Jesus' ministry:

> You know the message he sent to the people of Israel, *preaching peace* by Jesus Christ—he is Lord of all. That message spread throughout Judea, beginning in Galilee after the baptism that John announced: how God anointed Jesus of Nazareth with the Holy Spirit and with power; how he went about *doing good and healing all who were oppressed by the devil*, for God was with him. (emphasis added)

As Joel Green puts it, "Healing is pivotal for Jesus' identity and mission in the Gospel of Luke. Jesus' inaugural address tethers healing and teaching together as complementary means of proclaiming the good news" (Lk 4:16-30).[9] In the mission of the seventy, which prefigures the church's later mission to the Gentiles, the first word of address is "Peace be with you." If a "child of peace" is there, the door will be open; you shall enter, heal the sick and say, "The kingdom of God has come near to you" (Lk 10:9). If the peace is refused, it "shall return to you" and you shall wipe off the dust of your feet against them and say, "Yet know this: the kingdom of God has come near" (v. 11). Further, the seventy are "sent" (*apesteilen*), the same word used for Jesus' mission in Luke 4:18 and 43. Jesus sends out the seventy before his face (*pro prosōpou autou* [Lk 10:1]) to first cure the sick and then announce, "The kingdom of God has come near to you." While Luke's recurring verbal "proclaiming gospel" (*euangelizomai*) does not occur here, the announcement "Peace to this house!" introduces the gospel messenger. The house's peace response to Jesus' peace greeting is the condition for receiving healing and the kingdom of God.

---

[9]Green, "Healing," p. 759.

Luke's presentation of Jesus' reflective declaration on the mission of the seventy is most striking. First, Jesus speaks woes upon Chorazin and Bethsaida for failure to receive God's peace mission—God's *missio Dei* (Lk 10:13-16)—with words that echo the downfall of earlier self-exalted and oppressive kings (Is 14; Ezek 28):

> And you, Capernaum,
>> will you be exalted to heaven?
>> No, you will be brought down to Hades. (Lk 10:15)

Despite the extensive scope of rejection and judgment, Jesus *sees* also another result of the gospel of the kingdom's peace mission: "I watched [was seeing] Satan fall [falling] from heaven like a flash of lightning" (v. 18). Demons are expelled in the name of Jesus; a new reality dawns. Satan's rule ends; Jesus' reign begins! The victory has an even more enduring consequence in that "your names are written in heaven" (v. 20). The interrelated themes in Luke's gospel and healing emphases appear in this figure 3.1.

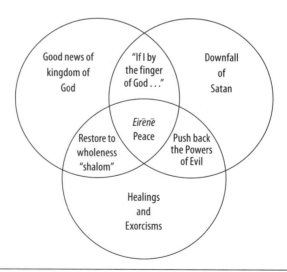

Figure 3.1. Peace and healing in Luke-Acts

One of Luke's special healing/deliverance stories occurs in Luke 13:10-17, the story of the bent-over woman (a good one to memorize and tell):

> Now he was teaching in one of the synagogues on the sabbath. And just

then there appeared a woman with a spirit that had crippled her for eighteen years. She was bent over and was quite unable to stand up straight. When Jesus saw her, he called her over and said, "Woman, you are set free from your ailment." When he laid his hands on her, immediately she stood up straight and began praising God. But the leader of the synagogue, indignant because Jesus had cured on the sabbath, kept saying to the crowd, "There are six days on which work ought to be done; come on those days and be cured, and not on the sabbath day." But the Lord answered him and said, "You hypocrites! Does not each of you on the sabbath untie his ox or his donkey from the manger, and lead it away to give it water? And ought not this woman, a daughter of Abraham whom Satan bound for eighteen long years, be set free from this bondage on the sabbath day?" When he said this, all his opponents were put to shame; and the entire crowd was rejoicing at all the wonderful things that he was doing.

This story, like others in Luke, portrays Jesus' power freeing people from bondage. Both Luke and Mark similarly portray Jesus as God's divine warrior come to vanquish evil, and set people free.[10] Numerous scholars identify here the exodus-liberation theme. Kathleen M. Fisher and Urban C. von Wahlde note that Mark chooses the four miracles of Mark 4:35–5:43 to show forth God's mighty power in Jesus' ministry. In the stilling of the storm "Jesus is acting in ways similar to Yahweh in recreating the harmony of the universe in reclaiming it from Satan." Then, in the exorcism of Mark 5:1-20 Jesus manifests divine power over personal possession by Satan. In the healing of the woman's incurable illness and in the raising of Jairus's daughter "the ultimate affliction of evil upon the world . . . is conquered." Further, they observe

that the miracles are not simply demonstrations of divine power but are exorcisms, the means by which, in Mark's apocalyptic world-view, God's sovereignty over Satan reasserts itself. And this sovereignty controls all areas of life. Thus Mark presents a Jesus who has power greater than any human malady, a power from God which exerts itself to right the order of creation by expelling and controlling Satan's grip over man and the world.[11]

---

[10]In Willard M. Swartley, *Covenant of Peace: The Missing Peace in New Testament Theology and Ethics* (Grand Rapids: Eerdmans, 2006), pp. 50-52, 112-20, I describe the relation between the Testaments on this theme of divine warrior and how it relates to peace and peacemaking.

[11]Kathleen M. Fisher and Urban C. von Wahlde, "The Miracles of Mark 4:35-5:43: Their Meaning and Function in the Gospel Framework," *Biblical Theology Bulletin* 11 (1981): 15.

Jesus' liberation is indeed comprehensive and complete. Mark depicts Jesus as God's warrior attacking Satan's stronghold in his exorcisms and healings as well. Jesus' method of subduing the enemy stands fully within the divine warfare, miracle tradition.[12] The word (of God) in and through Jesus is the power that smites the demons. In the Gospels the demons are violent and destructive, seeking injury and death of the human person;[13] Jesus' actions are liberating, restoring the human to tranquility and communion with self and others. In these confrontations history discloses the cosmic struggle of "Son of God versus demon, Holy Spirit versus unclean spirit." Jesus' purpose was "to enter this struggle on behalf of the true destiny of mankind and with his heavenly power . . . carry through to the victory, and to the life and communion that it brings."[14]

A difficult question arises: how much healing can we expect now and how much do we postpone until the final redemption of the body and the renewal of all creation (Rom 8:17-26)? Ray Anderson helpfully describes Jesus' ministry (in dealing with the Mt 8:17 citation of Isaiah 53:4: "He took our infirmities and bore our diseases"). He holds that Christ frees believers from the curse of the law (Gal 3:14; echo Deut 28), which includes diseases:

> Forgiveness of sins is a covenanted grace available as a spiritual reality to all in the present time, while healing of the body, as covenanted mercy promised in the eschaton through the resurrection, is only present in a provisional way, regardless of whether through miraculous intervention or through natural means.[15]

When the eschatological nature of both forgiveness of sin and bodily healing are affirmed, with both grounded in Jesus' resurrection *and* our promised resurrection, then we can say, yes, healing is indeed included

---

[12]Millard C. Lind's *Yahweh Is a Warrior* (Scottdale, Penn.: Herald Press, 1980) is a probing exposition of Yahweh's warfare as essentially miracle. True, many deviations from this model set forth in Ex 14:14 occur within Israel's history, but this does not change the essential nature of Yahweh's warfare.

[13]This does not mean that Jesus and the early Christians considered demons the cause of illness. Gary Ferngren contends that modern scholars who emphasize this point are wrong. For in both Christian and pagan texts a more positive view of physicians and (Hippocratic) medicine is evident during this period: *Medicine and Health Care in Early Christianity* (Baltimore: Johns Hopkins University Press, 2009).

[14]James Robinson, *The Problem of History in Mark* (London: SCM Press, 1957), pp. 39, 42.

[15]Ray S. Anderson, "Healing and the Atonement," unpublished paper, 1986.

within the atonement along with forgiveness of sin. Complete bodily healing awaits, however, eschatological fulfillment for its final consummation (Rom 8:17-26). While we glimpse now on occasion healing miracles, forgiveness of sins is God's present gift of grace in Jesus Christ (Eph 1:7; Col 1:14).

The theological fallacy of those who claim that immediate and full bodily healing is promised by God through the atonement is a failure to recognize that atonement, while enacted in the cross, is completed in the resurrection.

HEALING IN THE EARLY CHURCH

Jesus commissions and authorizes his apostles to heal the sick (Mt 10:1; Lk 10:9). The apostles and other early followers of Jesus continue that healing ministry. In Acts 8, 13 and 16, as the gospel moves into new geographical areas, Samaria, Cyprus, Asia Minor, it confronts the powers of evil and magic. The gospel overcomes those magical powers and opens the way for the gospel of the kingdom. Deliverance and healing flow together in Luke-Acts as standard signs of the good news of the *word* or *kingdom* of God (as in Acts 8:4-13 in describing Philip's ministry in Samaria and again in Luke's summary of Jesus' ministry in Acts 10:38). As God's Son, our Savior, Jesus comes into this world of oppression, sickness and brokenness to heal and make whole (Lk 4:18-19).

The first act of ministry in Acts is Peter's and John's dramatic healing of a lame man at the temple gate Beautiful (Acts 3:1-10). This healing leads to a continuing contest between the religious authorities, who accuse Jesus, and the apostles' defense focused on speaking and healing "in the name of Jesus" (Acts 3:6, 16; 4:10-12).[16] Later in Acts, Paul heals Eutychus, who fell out a window and was taken for dead (Acts 20:7-12).

In Paul's letters healing is identified as one of the gifts of the Spirit (*pneumatikoi*). In 1 Corinthians 12:8-10 both healing (*charismata iamatōn*) and discernment of spirits (*diakriseis pneumatōn*) are mentioned. In the summary of Paul's exhortation (vv. 28-30), the gift of healing recurs twice. While Acts narrates healing miracles of Paul, Paul himself in his letters doesn't mention such. Rather, he speaks of his own infirmity that he caus-

---

[16]Bonnie Thurston, *Spiritual Life in the Early Church* (Minneapolis: Fortress, 1993), pp. 34-43.

atively identifies as "a messenger of Satan to torment me." He "appealed to the Lord about this" three times that it would leave him, but the Lord's answer was, "My grace is sufficient for you, for power is made perfect in weakness" (2 Cor 12:7-9). This is important since it shows that healing does not occur in all cases, even for an apostle. This is surprising since the affliction is, by Paul's own perception, linked to an attack by a messenger (*angelos*) from Satan.[17] In Philippians 2:25-27 Paul mentions Epaphroditus who was "so ill that he nearly died." Then he says that "God had mercy on him," implying he was healed, apparently in a natural way, perhaps with medication.

The most frequently used New Testament text for the ongoing healing ministry in the church is James 5:14-15:

> Are any among you sick? They should call for the elders of the church and have prayer over them, anointing them with oil in the name of the Lord. The prayer of faith will save the sick, and the Lord will raise them up; and anyone who has committed sins will be forgiven.

This text has provided the basis for the church to practice healing ministry today in various ways. See chapter five for further treatment.

Of the many sources in the church fathers that speak to the church's continued healing ministry, I select quotes from Irenaeus and Origen. Denouncing the Gnostics, Irenaeus (A.D. c. 130-c. 200) says:

> For they can neither confer sight on the blind, nor hearing on the deaf, nor chase away all sorts of demons. . . . And so far are they from being able to raise the dead, as the Lord raised them, and the apostles by means of prayer, and as among the brotherhood oftentimes when necessity has arisen.[18]

Later Irenaeus speaks of the gifts of grace given to the disciples and the church, by which some drive out evil spirits, others "heal those who are sick by laying on their hands and make them whole."[19] He reiterates this as the mark of the true church whereas the leaders of the Gnostic sects have no such powers. The name of the Lord Jesus Christ, who truly lived among humans as a human and who also made all things, together with the gifts

---

[17]Wilkinson has an extended analysis of Paul's "thorn in the flesh" (*The Bible and Healing: A Medical and Theological Commentary* [Grand Rapids: Eerdmans, 1998], pp. 204-35).
[18]Irenaeus, *Adversus Haereses* 2.31.2, in *Exorcism and the Healing of the Sick*, trans. Reginald Maxwell Woolley (London: SPCK, 1932), p. 14.
[19]Ibid., 2.32.4, p. 15.

of the Spirit, mark the difference between Christ's true followers and the heretical Gnostics.

Origen (A.D. 185-254) also defends Christian belief against the pagans by his appeal to the healing and exorcist powers in the faith community:

> There are still preserved among Christians traces of the Holy Spirit which appeared in the form of a dove. They expel evil spirits and perform many cures and foresee certain events according to the will of the Logos. . . . The name of Jesus Christ can still remove distractions from the minds of men, expel demons, and also take away diseases.[20]

Other significant names associated with the healing tradition in the early church are Gregory Thaumaturgus (wonder-worker) narrated in writers Basil and Gregory of Nyssa. Martin of Tours was also known for his many healings.[21]

The exorcist dimension of healing played an important role in the early church. Everett Ferguson says of the early church's missionary success in the first three centuries:

> The most notable mark of the early church was its ability to deal with the spirit world in the Roman Empire. . . . I am persuaded that an important factor in the Christian success in the Roman world was the promise which it made of deliverance from demons.[22]

Ferguson observes that the early church fathers regarded Jesus' death and resurrection as the defeat of Satan.[23] Ferguson describes Irenaeus's view, saying, "By reason of his baptism, the Christian is delivered from the

---

[20]Origen, *Contra Celsus* 1.67; cf. ibid., 7.4.

[21]Secondary sources for further research on healing in the early church are Kelsey, *Healing and Christianity*, pp. 125-56; Ronald A. N. Kydd, *Healing Through the Centuries: Models for Understanding* (Peabody, Mass.: Hendrickson, 1998), pp. 70-81. An older work, Evelyn Frost, *Christian Healing* (London: A. R. Mowbray, 1940), is also helpful. Sources that document the continuing healing tradition in Eastern Orthodoxy are John T. Chirban, ed., *Health and Faith: Medical, Psychological, and Religious Dimensions* (Washington D.C.: University Press of America, 1991), and Stanley Samuel Harakas, *Health and Medicine in the Eastern Orthodox Tradition* (New York: Macmillan, 1990).

[22]Everett Ferguson, *Demonology of the Early Christian World* (New York: Edwin Mellen Press, 1984), pp. 129ff.

[23]For Irenaeus, e. g., "Christ's victory over the devil (is) the key motif in developing his doctrine of the atonement" (ibid., p. 124). The preaching of the gospel is the defeat of the demons. It brings the victory of Christ to bear upon the oppression here and now, and releases humans from Satan's tyranny.

power of demons and has been identified with Christ."[24] In many parts of the early Christian church catechetical preparation for baptism included daily priestly prayers expelling evil spirits. Baptism then culminated a person's exorcism. Since people came to the gospel from paganism, under the spell of the demons of the pagan religions, baptism was a rite of expelling the demon powers.

Concurring with Ramsay McMullen, Alan Kreider says that healing through exorcism was the chief factor in conversion, attracting people from the pagan world to Christianity because of its power over evil spirits. Kreider cites numerous sources from the fathers, with a report of a specific situation recounted by Origen: "Things like this lead many people to be converted to God, many to reform themselves, many to come to the faith."[25] Lutheran scholar Kyle Schiefelbein cites several prayers for the anointing with oil to heal the sick, including exorcism of evil (from *Apostolic Tradition*, c. A.D. 215, and Serapion, bishop in lower Egypt, c. A.D. 339-360). Sample lines are:

> May it [this oil] become to those who are anointed . . . a rejection of every disease and every sickness, for an amulet warding off every demon, for a departing of every evil spirit, . . . for a driving away of all fever and shiverings and every weakness, for good grace and forgiveness of sins, for a medicine of life and salvation, for health and wholeness of soul, body, spirit, for perfect strength (*Sacrament of Sarapion* 17).[26]

The waning of the early church healing/exorcistic practices came with the institutionalization of Christianity in the Constantinian church-state synthesis, though exceptions to this continued, with earlier fervency. The early church prayers of Serapion just cited, as well as the "anointing with oil," continued in the medieval Catholic Church and later in Lutheranism, according to Schiefelbein.[27] Though during the medieval and Reformation periods the healing and exorcist ministries became more liturgical and sacramental in expression, they continued to be practiced in

---

[24]Ibid., p. 125.

[25]Origen, cited in Alan Kreider, *The Change of Conversion and the Origin of Christendom* (Eugene, Ore.: Wipf & Stock, 2006), p. 17.

[26]Kyle K. Schiefelbein, "'Receive This Oil as a Sign of Forgiveness and Healing': A Brief History of the Anointing of the Sick and Its Use in Lutheran Worship," *Word & World* 30 (2010): 51.

[27]Ibid.

80   HEALTH, HEALING AND THE CHURCH'S MISSION

some areas of the Western and Eastern churches.[28]

During the medieval period the anointing with oil became a last rite for the dying. The Enlightenment and the rise of modern science further silenced the church in its healing ministry. Only recently, mostly through the influence of the Pentecostal and charismatic traditions, has healing become again a prominent practice in the church, and is now present in virtually all traditions, from Roman Catholic to evangelicals. Of this N. T. Wright writes:

> Recent times have seen a remarkable resurgence of a whole range of healing ministries. Twenty years ago, I doubt if you could have found a single book on, say, the healing of memories. Today there is likely to be a whole section in the average Christian bookshop, bringing together insights and experiences from an astonishingly wide range of people—monks, psychiatrists, lay workers, Orthodox, and Roman Catholics as well as Protestants and evangelicals.[29]

Several extensive studies of the healing in the church merit mention. Ronald Kydd's study of the historical relationship between Christianity and healing/health care focuses on *models* of Christian healing through the centuries. Compared to Avalos's description of the health care system of early Christianity (see chap. 8), many of the health care models of the later centuries (medieval and modern) became more complex and restrictive. Kydd describes these healing/health care models typologically:

- *confrontational*—early church, with modern representatives J. C. Blumhardt and John Wimber

- *intercessory*—saints on high, Brother André, Mary of Medjugorje

- *reliquirial*—bones of blessing, miracles as St. Médard

- *incubational*—Männendorf as place of mercy, message of Morija in persevering prayer

---

[28]This is especially true in connecting exorcism with baptism, evident in Henry Ansgar Kelly, *The Devil at Baptism: Ritual, Theology, and Drama* (Ithaca, N.Y.: Cornell University Press, 1985), a study of the history of the rites from the early church into the modern period. The baptismal liturgy of the Syrian Orthodox Church includes language of strong denunciation of the devil and evil spirits.

[29]N. T. Wright, *Bringing the Church to the World* (Minneapolis: Bethany House, 1992), pp. 132-33. For another brief assessment of healing in church history see Lewis B. Smedes, ed. *Ministry and the Miraculous: A Case Study at Fuller Theological Seminary* (Pasadena, Calif.: Fuller Theological Center, 1987), pp. 35-39.

- *revelational*—William Branham, Kathryn Kuhlman
- *soteriological*—Oral Roberts[30]

In the reliquirial model extensive travel was necessary to get to the holy relics that bestowed healing power through touch and adoration. In the incubational model long periods of waiting were common place. The other four models had less prohibitive factors; in the famous Blumhardt exorcism story the breakthrough came after several years of persistent confrontational prayer, at which time the departing demon shrieked, "Christ is Victor." Blumhardt (d. 1880) ministered to the sick in a Kurhaus (healing center) in Bad Boll, east of Stuttgart, Germany, for thirty years. He was also a dedicated competent pastor and theologian. Karl Barth names Blumhardt as one of his mentors.[31]

In the nineteenth century an emphasis on a passive, suffering response to illness prevailed, especially for women, whose suffering was understood to signify a sanctified life. This theological understanding, especially in the Reformed tradition, was "a passive resignation to afflictive providence."[32] The Lutheran tradition is ambivalent on anointing with oil to heal the sick. Luther himself said both yes and no; no to the Catholic reductionism of the practice to last rites, but yes for healing associated with the faith of the supplicant.[33] Olavus Petri, Luther's student, produced a manual that included such a rite in 1529. But no such rite appeared again in any Lutheran manual until Wilhelm Löhe's training manual for pastors and missionaries in the mid-nineteenth century. But again in the early twentieth century it disappeared in pastoral liturgy and practice. Then in 1958 a study committee recommended its use guardedly. In 1982 the Lutheran Book of Worship with its Occasional Service included "the first healing rite of its kind in Lutheran service books."[34] Much earlier, however, Methodist John Wesley emphasized "heal the sick" as a command of

---

[30]Kydd, *Healing Through the Centuries.*

[31]Ibid., pp. 34-45, for extended recounting of Blumhardt's ministry. Karl Barth mentions Blumhardt in the third movement of his doctrine of reconciliation: *Church Dogmatics*, vol. 4; part 3.1, *The Doctrine of Reconciliation*, trans. G. W. Bromiley (Edinburgh: T & T Clark, 1961), pp. 168-73.

[32]Heather Curtis, *Faith in the Great Physician: Suffering and Divine Healing in American Culture; 1860-1900* (Baltimore: Johns Hopkins University Press, 2007), p. 167.

[33]Schiefelbein, "Receive This Oil," pp. 55-59.

[34]Ibid., pp. 57-61.

Christ. He opened a health clinic and wrote a manual for good health.[35]

But this changed in official Methodism by the turn of the century with new emphases on "faith cure" in the holiness movement and then the Pentecostal movement succeeding it (particularly W. J. Seymour, A. J. Gordon, A. B. Simpson and Aimee Semple McPherson). The dramatic growth of Pentecostal churches in the last several decades flows from their emphases on the Holy Spirit and healing.[36] In the twentieth century new healing emphases emerged in virtually all church traditions. Kris Miller examines three main Protestant church traditions of healing and practice in the twentieth century: Anglican, Pentecostal and "Third Wave."[37] Mark Wenger examines the Mennonite practice of anointing with oil. Because of the misuse of this sacrament in Roman Catholicism in the sixteenth century, Anabaptists (forbears of Mennonites) spoke mostly against it. Among Mennonites, anointing with oil for healing began in the nineteenth and twentieth centuries, and continues into the present.[38]

Porterfield's extensive history of healing in Christianity recounts numerous types of healing that occurred globally during the modern period. Protestants tended to discount indigenous healing practices, while Catholics continued accommodation, blending the healing wisdom and practice of indigenous cultures with either Christian or medical healing practices of the time. Western people, however, continued to employ "spiritual practices for protection against the stresses of modernization, . . . in New England and Paris as well Maharasta and French Equatorial Africa."[39]

Adding to the ambiguity of the healing tradition during this period, *healing* became politicized, especially by liberal Protestants, for the gospel

---

[35]Sally Dyck, "Editorial: Stick to What We Know," *Circuit Rider* 34, no. 3 (2010): 1.

[36]See the issue of the *International Review of Mission* 93, nos. 370 and 371 (July-October 2004) devoted to "divine healing, pentecostalism, and mission," especially the articles "The Holy Spirit and the Church's Mission of Healing" by Norberto Saracco (pp. 413-20) and "The Spirit, Healing and Mission: An Overview of the Biblical Canon" by John Christopher Thomas (pp. 421-42).

[37]Kris A. Miller, "Streams of Healing: The Theological Frameworks of Prayer for Healing in Three Twentieth-Century Protestant Traditions" (unpublished thesis, Abilene, Tex.: Abilene Christian University, 2002).

[38]Mark R. Wenger, "Anointing the Sick with Oil in the Mennonite Church: An Exercise in Practical Theology" (unpublished dissertation, Richmond, Va.: Union Theological Seminary and Presbyterian School of Christian Education, 2000), pp. 43-48 (for Anabaptists); pp. 40-160 (for origins among Mennonites); and p. 119 (for an outline of a service for anointing).

[39]Amanda Porterfield, *Healing in the History of Christianity* (Oxford: Oxford University Press, 2005), p. 121.

witness focused mostly against social injustices: colonization, rich countries oppressing poor countries, and also protest against the depraved idol practices of the people they wished to convert. The missionaries cried out against the human misery of the people, but their doctrinaire interpretation of the gospel excluded consideration of positive benefit from indigenous practices of healing. Competitiveness between missionary groups, especially Protestant and Catholic, also clouded the healing gospel. "Tendencies to explain Christian theology in terms of social justice had important implications for conceptions of Christian healing. Advocates of social justice equated the healing power of Christ with the reconciliation that followed the defeat of sinful forces of oppression. This language of social justice harked back to the healing acts of Jesus . . . but the modern gospel of political liberation . . . reflected the politicization and secularization of modern Christian life."[40]

In this context of mission efforts new indigenous forms of Christian healing sprang up worldwide. Missionary historian Andrew Walls has cataloged the indigenous movements in Africa. Healing miracles played a dominant role in the growth, vitality and spawning of these movements. In sub-Saharan Africa, says Walls, "the Christian God is known by vernacular names. The relationship between Africa's old religion and its new one is cemented in the convention of speech."[41]

Colonial expansion in America had devastating health results for Native Americans. Great numbers died of new diseases brought by the European colonists: smallpox, influenza, measles, etc., Jesuit missionaries practiced Christian forms of healing and numerous accounts of healings were attributed to sacred rites and holy objects used in healing ceremonies. But the epidemics destroyed their healing credibility, resulting in Native American persecution of the Jesuits, forcing them into hiding.

An outstanding exception to this dismal landscape of mission efforts is the story of Kateri Tekakwitha (1656-1680), born to parents who died of smallpox. Her mother was Algonquin and her father, Mohawk. Because her parents had smallpox when she was born, she was crippled, disfigured and partially blind. Under the tutelage of Jesuit hospital nuns she was

---

[40]Ibid., pp. 123-24.
[41]Andrew F. Walls, *The Cross-Cultural Process in Christian History* (Maryknoll, N.Y.: Orbis, 2002), pp. 121-23; cited also by Porterfield, *Healing*, p. 125.

converted to Christianity and became a suffering saint, even an ascetic, flagellating herself to identify fully with the sufferings of Christ. She remained celibate and dedicated her life to devotion to the Blessed Mary. In her sufferings she became "a powerful symbol of the plight of her people. In her application of suffering toward spiritual and charitable ends, she represented the heroism of her people, as well as the Virgin's powerful sorrow for the sufferings of her son." Beatified in 1980, she has now been adopted by virtually all Native Americans, with healing effect influencing various tribes to work together for their common welfare.[42]

Other important Christian healers emerged in Native American history: Handsome Lake, an Iroquois (c. 1745-1815), and Wovoka, a Paiute Indian, known in English circles as Jack Wilson. Lake grew up amid his "demoralized, impoverished, and disease-stricken people" and had visions of heaven and hell, about which the missionaries preached. In his visions he saw "two roads in the spirit world, one leading to the house where Indians who succumbed to the vices of the white man were punished for their sins, and the other to a land of abundant fields and streams where faithful Indians lived in robust health." Lake also received a Moses-type law code for his people, known as *Gai'wiio* or "The Good Message." Renouncing sin and recovering health are motifs in both this behavioral code and Lake's entire ministry.[43]

Wovoka grew up in a Presbyterian family. His healing ministry came through a powerful vision in 1889. He saw his beloved native people in heaven, healed and well, along with some white people. This empowered him for a lifetime mission of healing as a shaman among his people. He preached fervently for natives and whites to get along with each other and live peacefully together. He is known for his founding of the Ghost Dance, in which some participants during this circle dance "fell to the ground and experienced visions of their deceased relatives in heaven." As a ministry of healing and reconciliation, he received numerous delegations to his home in Nevada, from Ute, Shoshone, Arapahoe, Cheyenne, Sioux, Bannock and Mohave tribes.[44]

Black Elk also was a healing figure. He helped to recreate the Sun

---

[42]Porterfield, *Healing*, pp. 127-28.
[43]Ibid., p. 129.
[44]Ibid., pp. 129-30.

Dance, in which "individuals found help with alcoholism and other forms of disease, failure, and misfortune. They also found well-being through identification with a traditional religious community, as did the family members and friends who gathered to support them." Healing of various types resulted from his ministry. In *The Sacred Pipe*, Elk "laid out the meaning and therapeutic benefits of the seven rituals sacred to Oglala Sioux, much as a catechism might introduce readers to the seven sacraments of the Catholic Church."[45]

In assessing these healers and their contribution, we value their blend of Christian faith with native traditions. The test for a valid synthesis is whether or not they affirm Jesus as Savior, Healer and Lord. The healing ministry of Jesus and the church through the centuries challenges us to approach human need holistically, refusing to dichotomize material/physical and spiritual/moral needs. It also means that we as Christian believers are called to see ourselves as healers and recognize this as a vital part of Christian ministry. As such we will live in openness to the presence of God's kingdom, praying for holistic healing, including the miraculous, but not in such a way that we exalt or condemn ourselves, or define God by *our* faith or lack of it.

Fred Pratt Green's hymn text magnifies Christ as healer:

O Christ, the healer, we have come
To pray for health, to plead for friends,
How can we fail to be restored
When reached by love that never ends?

From every ailment flesh endures
Our bodies clamor to be freed,
Yet in our hearts we would confess
That wholeness is our deepest need.

In conflicts that destroy our health
We recognize the world's disease;
Our common life declares our ills,
Is there no cure, O Christ, for these?

Grant that we all, made one in faith,
In your community may find

---

[45]Ibid., pp. 131-32 (quote on p. 131).

The wholeness that, enriching us,
Shall reach the whole of humankind.[46]

EXCURSUS

Porterfield describes several healers in global cultures. I cite three different strands: the first both laudable and abhorrent; the second and third, exemplary:

1. China: Liang Afa. In 1832 Liang was the first Chinese convert to Protestant Christianity. In 1836 he wrote his own account of the Christian faith. On reading this book, Hong Xiuquan became an influential convert. Proclaiming himself to be the younger brother of Jesus, he began baptizing, preaching and healing. His followers, known as God Worshipers, "mushroomed into a mass movement after 1842, at the end of the Opium War. . . . [Most unfortunately,] Hong's movement developed into an organized political and military force that took hold of China's economic heartland with ruthless force." Millions of people died in the revolution; Hong then founded the new Taiping (Heavenly Kingdom) dynasty in 1853. The movement "had a chilling effect on reverence for Daoist deities," smashing temples and exorcising "Daoist deities as malevolent demons." Though he was a Christian miracle healer, Hong's Taiping revolution had disastrous results. What a tragedy, trying to establish God's kingdom through military might. In 1864 the Taiping dynasty ended, destroyed by Qing troops.[47]

2. Africa: Liberian William Wade Harris (1865-1929). Through a vision Harris declared himself to be son and prophet of God, called to a mission of bringing many people to the gospel. A charismatic figure wearing a white robe with black bands, he danced with a "gourd rattle to ward off evil spirits. He admonished people to give up their old gods and reliance on traditional healers and baptized more than a hundred thousand people before being expelled from the Ivory Coast in 1914 by French officials." His converts accepted the Methodist missionaries in 1924, and his influence spread throughout West Africa, with many Harrist churches

---

[46]Fred Pratt Green, "O Christ, the Healer, We Have Come" (1969). Used by permission from © Hope Publishing Co., Inc.
[47]Porterfield, *Healing*, pp. 133-34, supplemented by conversation with mission historian Wilbert Shenk.

flourishing. Later, a split occurred with some becoming Methodists and Catholics, and others remaining Harrist.[48]

3. South Africa (political healing). In South Africa traditional African spiritual healing practices fused with Marian devotion and Pentecostal Spirit gifts generated and inspired a distinctive African religious leadership that guided the people to a nonviolent end to apartheid's many injustices and killings. Mvumbi Luthuli (1898-1967), educated at Protestant schools, headed the first generation of leaders, with Nelson Mandela and Desmond Tutu leading the second and current generation. Mandela, the first black democratically elected president, appointed Tutu to head the Truth and Reconciliation Commission, forging a "healing of relationships" and healing festering wounds.[49]

---

[48]Ibid., pp. 134-37. For an extensive analysis of the Harris movement, see David A. Shank, "A Prophet of Modern Times: The Thought of William Wade Harris" (unpublished Ph.D. diss., Aberdeen, U.K.: Aberdeen University, 1980).

[49]Porterfield, *Healing*, pp. 137-40.

4

❖

Biblical and Theological
Analysis of Healing

As Christians, if we are to love as Jesus loved, we must first come to terms with suffering. Like Jesus, we simply cannot be cool and detached from our fellow human beings. Our years of living as Christians will be years of suffering for and with other people. Like Jesus, we will love others only if we walk with them in the valley of darkness—the dark valley of moral dilemmas, the dark valley of oppressive structures and diminished rights.

Joseph Cardinal Bernardin, *The Gift of Peace*

Reflecting on the biblical and theological issues of healing leads us to think paradoxically. At least four paradoxes or dialectical relationships emerge. Or we might wish to think of these as tensions or mysteries. In daily experience we often think of these in either-or terms, not interactive perspectives. Our questions find only partial answers. We are thrown back, on the one hand, to our finitude and limits, and on the other, we are determined to do something, at least to cope with the down side, or in our better moments to celebrate the goodness of life even in the midst of pain, anger and sadness.

Only as we see truth in paradox, as a mystery beyond ourselves, do we live fruitfully with the biblical imagery and theology of healing. Four paradoxes confront us:

1. *Humans are frail and finite, yet powerful as cocreators in the divine image.* We noted earlier Waldemar Janzen's analysis of the human being: we

must take account of our human frailty and vulnerability, and our potential as God's image bearers.

The relevance of this for any healing ministry is soon recognized. We empathize with our brother or sister whom we desire to be healed when we see him or her as lowly, needy and vulnerable. This condition arises partly from God's original design in making humans from the dust and partly by perversion of God's original design through human sin, which theologically we call the Fall. In light of these combined situations this view of human nature is more relevant to healing than lofty references to human dignity, reason, freedom, creativity, potentiality, gifts and even the often cited "image of God."[1]

We also noted how frequently psalms emphasize the frailty and finitude of our human existence. Job felt this frailty amid the cacophony of circumstances that engulfed his life. We too live with handicaps, disability, limitations and mortality. Given these realities, we may wonder if we are pawns in a master chess game whose players not only use us for their larger ends but even change the rules to make our anxieties about our own demise more unbearable and our waiting more excruciating.

But, yes, there is the other side of the paradox as well. We are created "in the image of God." As the psalmist puts it, we are "little lower than God" (variant reading, "angels") (Ps 8:5). In the Genesis narrative we are given the capacity for dominion over the earth. We can think, speak, remember and plan for the future.

Add to this our Christian belief about the human situation. Jesus, as the truly human Son of God and Son of Man, shows us the way to be truly human, created anew in the image of God. Jesus, in his true obedience to his Father, battled against the forces of evil that negatively play upon human frailty and finitude. He emerged Victor, inviting us to be heirs of that victory. Consequently, bleakness about the human condition is not the final word: rather God's transcendent power, love and glory come to us through Jesus Christ, our hope and empowerment. We are called to be image of God in this world; in Christ it is not only a call but a possibility (Eph 4:24–5:2).

This is the first paradox, a dialectical tension, yes, a mystery. Examples

---

[1]Waldemar Janzen, "Human Wholeness in Biblical Perspective," in *Still in the Image: Essays in Biblical Theology and Anthropology* (Newton, Kans.: Faith and Life Press, 1982), pp. 62-63.

of "God's creative and transforming power" at work are present in many communities and people: in the L'Arche communities, in Joseph Cardinal Bernardin's personal reflections as a cancer sufferer, in Joni Eareckson Tada's testimonies, and more. These are stories of human courage and divine grace, finding wholeness which may be healing from sickness or disability, or freedom in sickness to live life with purpose and fulfillment. On this latter point Marva Dawn speaks from experience and theology on *Being Well When We're Ill: Wholeness and Hope in Spite of Infirmity.*[2]

The most extensive presentation of this paradox shines through Paul's letters to the Corinthians. As Krister Stendahl cogently argues, physical infirmity is for Paul *weakness*, not sin. Further, this weakness is not a count against Paul or the power of the gospel. Rather, it identifies Paul with Christ; this weakness is "part and parcel of Paul's deepest religious experience" and stands at the center of his "theology of the cross."[3] Stendahl cites Paul's diagnosis of the human condition in Romans 5:6-10 (*weak, sinners* and *enemies* of God); in 2 Corinthians 12:9 Paul regards *weakness* not as a condemnation for sin or enmity. It is not a stain on his conscience. The weakness throws into bold relief the transcendent empowerment of our "earthen vessels" (2 Cor 4:6-10). Paul contrasts himself to the super-apostles and their self-authentication rooted in their inherent superior spiritual power and wisdom (2 Cor 11–12). This theology magnifies the paradox, for when we know and own our weakness, we are empowered by the promise, "My grace is sufficient for you" (2 Cor 12:9).[4]

The second paradox and mystery is an extension of the first.

2. Our human experience in this world knows incredible pain, suffering and anguish of spirit as a result of many natural and moral evils, but our experience in this world knows also an incomprehensible power of a loving God, a God who is healer and whose Son manifested that divine presence by "preaching the gospel of the kingdom and healing every disease and every infirmity among the people."

I illustrate the first part of the paradox of pain, suffering and anguish by referring to my brother Clifford, who, born with limited intellectual capacity, could never get beyond the fifth grade in school. One day when

---

[2]Marva Dawn, *Being Well When We're Ill: Wholeness and Hope in Spite of Infirmity* (Minneapolis: Augsburg, 2008).
[3]Krister Stendahl, *Paul Among Jews and Gentiles* (Philadelphia: Fortress, 1976), p. 47.
[4]Ibid., pp. 48-50.

crossing the road on his bicycle in front of our farm house to enter our lane, he did not see an oncoming car, was hit, then drug 150 feet under the car and ended up in a fetal position with his back under the transmission. No one expected him to live, but he did. Six years later another brother, Kenneth, lost control of a jack-knifed tractor and manure spreader on a slippery hill in our meadow on a sun-warmed January day. He was crushed to death by the overturned tractor.

Our collective stories, along with those appearing daily in our newspapers, highlight the magnitude of human pain in this world, compounding our human anguish and suffering. Listen to the complaint of the psalmist, arising out of the depths of his or her human anguish. Psalm 38 voices the pathos of human suffering. Experiences of suffering, of many different types, permeate the biblical narrative. In a combined Old and New Testament study of suffering, Erhard Gerstenberger and Wolfgang Schrage describe the range of experience: loss of a loved person or valued property, personal honor, or illness; violence; fear; failure and meaninglessness. These experiences are interpreted differently: as a curse for an evil deed, expiation of sin, divine punishment or discipline, educational value, satanic action, or the inscrutable purpose of God. Reactions to suffering include flight, immobility, active resistance, sublimation in the rational life, ritual defense, transformation of it into positive meaning and even perception that it reshapes the world.[5]

What is God's answer to Job? Is Job's righteousness vindicated in the final reversal of his fortune? Perhaps, but more to the main point of his agony over loss of family and health is his persistence in faithfulness as "servant of the Lord," in his sealed voiceless lips before the inexplicable.[6] As Christians we believe in a vindication of the suffering righteous in the world to come. In the "now" time, we identify with God's pathos, God's own suffering with the sufferers. In his outstanding book *The Prophets*, Abraham Heschel speaks of God's pathos in suffering for his people, drawing on Hosea and other prophets.

[5]Erhard S. Gerstenberger and Wolfgang Schrage, *Suffering* (Nashville: Abingdon, 1980), pp. 22-129.
[6]See Susan F. Mathews's essay on Job, "All for Naught: My Servant Job," in *The Bible and Suffering: Social and Political Implications*, ed. Anthony J. Tambasco (Mahweh, N.J.: Paulist Press, 2001), pp. 51-71. The narrative is framed by identifying Job as "my servant Job" (1:8; 2:3 and 42:7-8 [4x]).

Terence Fretheim's extensive study on suffering in the Old Testament emphasizes God is not external to the world but internally related, suffering with the covenant people and even all creation. Three chapters of *The Suffering of God* focus on God's presence with us in suffering. First (chap. 7), God suffers *because* of broken covenant relationship, Israel's idolatries and human resistance to God. In the "memory of God" the past and the present collide so that Hosea and Jeremiah describe the sufferings of the present in relation to past (un)faithfulness. The lament psalms express God's and peoples' suffering in the present and often in relation to the past. Fretheim cites numerous texts (e.g., Is 1:2-3; Jer 2:29-32) that voice this suffering, which is what Heschel and Fretheim call the *pathos of God:* "Memory intensifies the painfulness of the present as God struggles over what shape the people's future should take" (Jer 5:7-9; 9:7, 9).[7]

Second (chap. 8), God suffers and mourns *with* the people's suffering in Israel's bondage (Ex 2:23-25; 3:7-8) and later impending exile (Is 54:7-8). Israel's plight evokes language of mourning and compassion more than lament and accusation. Many texts are "divine funerary laments" (Ezek 2:10; 26:17-18, to cite a few).[8]

Third (chap. 9), God suffers *for* the people. Sacrifices enact the reality of the divine suffering, as sign of restoring relationship. But these do not annul the suffering (Is 43:23-24; cf. 1 Pet 2:24 where Christ bears the sins of many). "Look[ing] on the one whom they have pierced" depicts God's and Christ's suffering *for* the sins of the people (Zech 12:10, quoted in Jn 19:37).[9] "God and prophet enter into the mourning of the people" (Jer 4:19; 8:18–9:1—"My grief is beyond healing," RSV).[10] Hosea 6:4-6 and 11:8-9 ("Your love is like a morning cloud" yet "How can I give you up") poignantly express the pathos of God's sufferings. God's suffering (*because of, with* and *for* us) assures us that God does not forget us in our sufferings, personally and corporately. God is present in the finitude and frailty of our human experience, including sickness.

Jung recognizes this in his *Answer to Job*, Jesus as sufferer is God's an-

---

[7]Terence E. Fretheim, *The Suffering of God: An Old Testament Perspective* (Philadelphia: Fortress, 1989), p. 122.
[8]Ibid., pp. 130-36.
[9]Ibid., pp. 138-46.
[10]Ibid., p. 160

swer.[11] He bears our infirmities—both *with* us and *for* us. God is as much related to the suffering side of this paradox as to the victory side. Hospice chaplains and nurses know this experientially: terminal illness, death and dying are a part and culmination of living. Only when one harbors resentment and fails to filter the wrongs in life with words and acts of forgiveness is suffering altogether sorrowful and without hope of vindication.

Daniel Patte, in his study of Paul's faith convictions, points out that the believers' basic identity and foremost certification as Christian is in and through suffering (1 Thess 1:6-7). In this experience they are imitators (*mimētai)* of Jesus Christ; in this they knew and we know who we are. In this they became an example (*typos)* to others.[12]

Now we shift to the other side of the paradox. We know also a powerful and loving God, a God who comes to us as helper and healer, savior and victor. The story of biblical faith is a story of deliverance out of troubles; the Lord God is redeemer of the oppressed, comforter of the sufferer. The description of God and Jesus as healer permeates the biblical narrative and is close to the center of our Christian faith and hope.

Even within this affirmation of God as healer, there arises another paradox, a mystery. In one sense all sickness arises from sin and evil; sickness compromises the goodness of creation, the paradise which God originally created for humans. As Karl Barth put it, sickness is "like death itself, unnatural and disorderly, an element in the rebellion of chaos against God's creation, and an act and declaration of the devil and demons."[13] Nicholas Wolterstorff voices a similar protest, as he faced the tragic death of his son at age twenty-five, "Death is awful, demonic. . . . To comfort me, you have to come close. Come sit beside me on my mourner's bench."[14] After crying out to God in the tradition of the lament psalms and refusing easy answers, Wolterstorff says, "I cannot fit it all together at all. I can only, with Job, endure. I do not know why God did not prevent Eric's death. To live without an answer is precarious. It's hard to keep one's footing."[15] Again, in his poetic reflections on his son's death, Wolterstorff

---

[11]Carl Jung, *Answer to Job* (Princeton, N.J.: Princeton University Press, 1973).

[12]Daniel Patte, *Paul's Faith and the Power of the Gospel* (Philadelphia: Fortress, 1983), pp. 134-39.

[13]Karl Barth, cited in Klaus Seybold and Ulrich B. Mueller, *Sickness and Healing* (Nashville: Abingdon, 1978), p. 192.

[14]Nicholas Wolterstorff, *Lament for a Son* (Grand Rapids: Eerdmans, 1987), p. 34.

[15]Ibid., p. 67. Hartzler has good insights on suffering in the context of lament (Rachel Nafziger

succinctly speaks, "Instead of explaining our suffering, God shares it."[16] This emphasis is central to Jürgen Moltmann's theology of suffering also. For Moltmann, the cross is at the center of Christian theology, indeed the route to hope.[17]

Catastrophes, like Wolterstorff's son's death when mountain climbing, illnesses like AIDS, the horrific human suffering from war, plagues, earthquakes, tsunamis, floods and especially children's deaths—a theme in Stanley Hauerwas's treatment of the inadequacy of any theodicy (shared also by Wolterstorff)—lack explanation.[18] No philosophical theodicy satisfies. None resolves how a good, all-powerful God can allow bad things to happen to "good people."[19] God in Christ suffers with us, bears the cross

---

Hartzler, *Grief and Sexuality: Life after Losing a Spouse* [Scottdale, Penn.: Herald Press, 2006], pp. 37-51).

[16]Wolterstorff, *Lament for a Son*, p. 81.

[17]Jürgen Moltmann, *The Crucified God: The Cross of Christ as the Foundation and Criticism of Christian Theology* (New York: Harper & Row, 1974), pp. 64-65; 152-53, 204-16; cf. his *The Way of Jesus Christ: Christology in Messianic Dimensions* (Minneapolis: Fortress Press, 1993), pp. 151-212.

[18]Deanna A. Thompson, religion teacher at Hamlin University in St. Paul, Minnesota, writes from "the heart" on this topic. Battling stage four cancer she normally finds the classroom a "cancer-free zone." But as they approach the topic of suffering and theodicy, unlike her usual pedagogy, she hesitates to connect the discussion with personal disclosure. Some students propose God sends the "hard times" of trials and suffering to make us stronger, to build character. She asks, "But do the hard times always lead to growth?" The room falls silent. She then discloses her cancer plight, acknowledging that some people told her God sent the cancer to make her a stronger person. But, she says, "I don't buy it. Living with cancer sucks, frankly, and I have a hard time believing in a God who sends people cancer or other terminal illness to teach them a lesson. This view simply does not acknowledge the full scope of suffering that pervades many of our lives." She begins to shake and knows she can go no further with personal disclosure, so as teachers do she redirects the discussion, "Why might those who suffer find this view of God and suffering inadequate?" ("Suffering Through Lent," *Christian Century*, March 22, 2011, pp. 12-13). She connects this to Jesus' suffering: God did not make Jesus suffer to teach him a lesson. Rather, Jesus as revealer of God shows God is with us in our suffering. God suffers *with* those who suffer. God also promises death and destruction are not the end. Crushing natural evils like earthquakes and tsunamis raise even harder theodicy questions.

[19]Harold Kushner's construal of the problem in popular vein in *When Bad Things Happen to Good People*—that we are forced to choose between a "good" God or an "all-powerful God"—misses the heart of the biblical story: God in divine goodness is present in the cross and is also powerfully present in the resurrection. A biblical construal of this problem portrays God as first and foremost a God of *love*, which at the heart of the narrative shatters the choice between "good" and "all-powerful." John Goldingay's excellent treatment of suffering in his *Old Testament Theology* identifies several points of clash between our modern, Western questions about suffering and the Old Testament's view of suffering. Rather than complain about why bad things happen to good people, the question is: Why does God allow the wicked to prosper and oppress the poor? Those who pen the Scripture identify with sufferers, even to the point of "accepting suffering as a vocation" and valuing most of all "relationship with God," come what may (*Old Testament Theology, Volume 3: Israel's Life* [Downers Grove, Ill.: IVP Academic, 2009], p. 695; see pp. 681-99).

and calls the faith community to care for the suffering, while not making suffering a virtue to be desired. Hauerwas eloquently says, "historically, Christians have not had a 'solution' to the problem of evil [or suffering]. Rather, they have had a community of care that has made it possible for them to absorb the destructive terror of evil that constantly threatens to destroy all human relations."[20]

In his helpful book *Is God to Blame?* Gregory Boyd rejects "pat answers" to suffering that stem often from a "blueprint worldview," which holds that even the most horrible tragedy accords with God's will and purpose. He counters the "blueprint" view with God's warfare against evil, culminating in the suffering Christ on our behalf,

> The cross reveals that God's omnipotence is displayed in self-sacrificial love, *not sheer might*. God conquers sin and the devil not by a sovereign decree but by a wise and humble submission to crucifixion. In doing this, the cross reveals God's omnipotence is not primarily about control but about his compelling love. God conquers evil and wins the heart of people by self-sacrificial love, not by coercive force.[21]

Human freedom is also at stake. Joni Eareckson Tada, suffering many years from quadriplegia and now coming to terms with breast cancer, sees God's mercy evident in human suffering. In the context of the fall of humans into sin, she says, "Suffering is connected to sin; if God were to get rid of suffering, he'd have to get rid of sin, and then he'd have to get rid of sinners—and God is too merciful to do that."[22] Advancement of the gospel is greater than miracle![23]

The Gospels present the cross as God's supreme revelation of love, the great miracle of the gospel. Out of the ashes of suffering and death come

---

[20]Stanley Hauerwas, *Naming the Silences: God, Medicine, and the Problem of Suffering* (Grand Rapids: Eerdmans, 1990), p. 53. Hauerwas approvingly cites John Douglas Hall's critique of Kushner's *When Bad Things Happen to Good People*, saying that it is not God's goodness that is at issue but the biblical story, which from beginning to end is one of "love, sheer love, that constitutes the basis of . . . the relation between the principal characters. . . . Because Kushner fails to grasp (or at least express this), his response to . . . human suffering, while full of practical insights, is theologically and humanly unsatisfying" (Hauerwas, *Naming the Silences*, p. 57).

[21]Gregory A. Boyd, *Is God to Blame? Beyond Pat Answers to the Problem of Suffering* (Downers Grove, Ill.: InterVarsity Press, 2003), p. 49.

[22]"Joni Eareckson Tada on Something Greater Than Healing," interview by Sarah Pulliam Bailey, *Christianity Today*, October 8, 2010, p. 32.

[23]Ibid., p. 30.

resurrection and hope. This is paradoxical. On the one hand, the cross is the victory of malevolence: religious leaders collude across party lines to accuse Jesus and cry "crucify." Pilate, the empire's face, drives the nails into Jesus' hands and feet, and Satan rejoices. This despicable crucifixion is the devil's glory. On the other hand, it is God's opportune moment to intervene, to raise Jesus from death, to dismay the religious leaders, taunt the power of the empire, and trump Satan's strategies. In John's Gospel Jesus' self-giving love culminates in his being "lifted up" on the cross. This is his glorification. Only through this paradox can Calvary be a fulfillment of God's salvation purpose. The cross demonstrates God's unfailing love for the sufferer. In turn, the community of the cross exists in its solidarity with suffering.

The Christian's hope lies indeed in the healing work of the suffering Christ: "He took our infirmities [or sicknesses] and bore our diseases." Matthew cites this from Isaiah's fourth suffering servant song (Mt 8:17; cf. Is 53:4) in the middle of his ten healing miracles (Mt 8–9; cf. Mt 15:29-31). By his chastisement we are made whole: we receive shalom (Is 53:5). In Christ's servant suffering—and ours—the mystery of this paradox finds some resolution, but only some. We continue to await the redemption of our bodies, when all creation's groaning will be consummated by the new heavens and the new earth in which only righteousness will dwell, from which evil and sickness will be banished forever. In living with this paradox of Christ's suffering and victory, and the horrible suffering that continues in history, we face keenly the "now, not yet" tension in Christian experience and hope. Biblical faith offers us apocalyptic hope, which envisions a coming world free of suffering. Our tears are wiped away and sorrow and sickness are no more (Rev 21:4). Children play in the streets without danger (Zech 8:5) and the tree of life is healing for the nations (Rev 22:2).

We know that now "we have this treasure in earthen vessels, to show that the transcendent power belongs to God and not to us" (1 Cor 4:7 RSV). It is precisely because of this tension between receiving the transcendent power and knowing it does not belong to us that the apostle Paul can say, "We are afflicted in every way, but not crushed; perplexed, but not driven to despair; persecuted but not forsaken; struck down, but not destroyed; always carrying in the body the death of Jesus; so that the life of Jesus may also be made visible in our bodies" (2 Cor 4:8-10).

When faced with heart-rending and inexplicable suffering, we can learn from Job, who trusts God even when the explanations of his would-be comforters ring hollow. In the end he covers his mouth; he knows he cannot fathom God. He can only persevere in the covenant love relationship. As Hauerwas puts it in describing the function of the lament psalms,

> The psalms of lament do not simply reflect our experience; they are meant to form our experience of despair. They are meant to name the silences that our suffering has created. They bring us into communion with God and one another, communion that makes it possible to acknowledge our pain and suffering, to rage that we see no point to it, and yet our very acknowledgment of that fact makes us a people capable of living life faithfully. We are able to do so because we know that the God who has made our life possible is not a God merely of goodness and power, but the God whom we find manifested in the calling of Israel and the life, cross, and resurrection of Jesus of Nazareth.[24]

By "living life faithfully" in and through the lament, the sufferer opens the wounded self to new life, even beauty and joy, as Hartzler aptly says:

> When an individual or community suffers or enters into the suffering of others and utters laments to God from that place of suffering, the individual or community can begin to experience the inklings of joy in the midst of sorrow and glimpses of beauty in the rubbish of grief. Eventually, authentic thanksgiving and praise can be raised to God.[25]

Some years ago I spoke at Philhaven Hospital in eastern Pennsylvania and addressed the suffering of mental illness. A counselor, Rev. Cornel Rempel, gave me "nine maxims" on this difficult topic. I have found these helpful.[26]

---

[24]Hauerwas, *Naming the Silences*, p. 82. The topic of human suffering is discussed biblically and philosophically in the numerous essays in Jan Lambrecht and Raymond F. Collins, ed., *God and Human Suffering*, Louvain Theological and Pastoral Monographs 3 (Grand Rapids: Eerdmans, 1990). See also the insightful essay by Marcus A. Gigliotti on Ecclesiastes, "Qoheleth: Portrait of an Artist in Pain," in *The Bible and Suffering*, ed. Anthony J. Tambasco (Mahweh, N.J.: Paulist Press, 2002), pp. 72-92.

[25]Hartzler, *Grief and Sexuality*, p. 55.

[26]Used with permission from Cornel Rempel, director of pastoral services and clinical pastoral education (CPE) supervisor at Philhaven, Penn. (currently living in Winnipeg, Manitoba, Canada).

Suffering is not God's desire for us,
but occurs in the process of life.

Suffering is not given in order to teach us something,
but through it we learn.

Suffering is not given to us to teach others something,
but through it they may learn.

Suffering is not given to punish us,
but is sometimes the consequence of sinful acts or poor judgment.

Suffering does not occur because our faith is weak,
but through it our faith may be strengthened.

Suffering does not mean that God depends on it to achieve his purposes,
but through it his purposes are sometimes achieved.

Suffering is not always to be avoided at all costs,
but is sometimes willingly endured for redemptive purposes.

Suffering may either destroy us—
or contribute to significant meaning in life.

The will of God has more to do with how we respond to life,
than with how life deals with us.

Wuellner expresses a similar view:

> One thing we definitely know. God has not deliberately sent tragedy and suffering upon us. Though they are allowed, endured by God, they are not God's *intention* for us. Not once in the Gospels does Jesus say that God sends tragedy and pain either to test us or to punish us. . . . [T]he New Testament makes clear that God is *always* on the side of healing, release, and reconciliation.[27]

For essays on and stories of suffering, reflecting both the human agony and the hope of faith, see the sixteen short, insightful essays on suffering in an issue of *Vision*.[28]

3. We know the power of our own egoisms, our angers, our hatred of enemies, our emptiness, our loneliness and at times our feelings of low or no self-worth,

---

[27]Flora Slosson Wuellner, *Prayer, Fear, and Our Powers: Finding Our Healing, Release, and Growth in Christ* (Nashville: Upper Room, 1989), p. 62.
[28]Gayle Gerber Koontz, ed., *Vision: A Journal for Church and Theology* 8, no. 2 (Fall 2007).

but we know also community of the Spirit as loving, caring, as koinonia, rooted in a faith, hope and love that enables us to transcend our sin and hopelessness.

This third paradox riddles our human experience. To illustrate the plight and trap of our human egoisms and loneliness, I quote Jean Vanier, whose description focuses on the suffering and needs of handicapped, but also, as he says at the outset of his essays, embraces the experience of all humans to lesser or greater degrees:

> In all our communities we have witnessed the deep suffering of handicapped people. So many have felt that they were (and are) a disappointment and a burden for their parents. So many have felt the pangs of loneliness and anguish coming from rejection and despisement. So many have been closed up in institutions. They come to us with terribly broken images of themselves; they feel devalued and useless; there is no meaning to their lives. Inside them there is fear and, frequently, concealed anger towards themselves and others. Many have touched the very depths of despair. . . .
>
> Each one carried his or her secret hurts. . . .
>
> And those secret hurts incite them often to lose trust in themselves: either they close in upon themselves or they play the clown, or else they may become aggressive, or hide sometimes in a world of dreams. They have no hope. . . .
>
> The need to be loved and cherished is so fundamental to every human being. If we feel we are not wanted, are considered useless and a burden, we close ourselves up and harden ourselves in order to avoid suffering the pangs of loneliness and anguish. Then we do things to prove our worth to ourselves and others, or perhaps we become angry when faced with the apparent "worthlessness" of others or ourselves. We can become drunk with desire to be efficacious or to dominate, to prove, to be a success. But still our hearts yearn deeply for this personal relationship, for somebody who will understand us, love and cherish us, accept us as we are, and see in us, deeper than our limits, the meaning of our lives.[29]

Popular books on Christian psychology often address anger, depression, emptiness, loneliness and low self-esteem. We find these feelings not only in others but also in ourselves; we know existentially the dark side of this paradox. We may even join Job and the psalmist in crying out to God to vindicate us in our alienation and despair.

---

[29]Jean Vanier, "L'Arche: Its History and Vision," in *The Church and Disabled Persons*, ed. Griff Hogan (Springfield, Ill.: Templegate, 1983), pp. 54-55.

But we know also the transforming hope and empowerment of Christian faith. We know meaning, purpose and joy in life that arises from community and worship. These too are experiences that Christian believers frequently and commonly share. Indeed, these are often most evident among the handicapped, the poor and the oppressed, and certainly among all of us when we are truly penitent, humble and trustful of God's purpose and presence in our lives. We know the empowerment of praise and thanksgiving that accompany the worshiping community filled with faith, hope and love. We know that love supersedes suffering and never ends. Eric Segal's *Love Story* witnesses to the joyful mystery: when we reach out to others in love, even in the midst of our own pain and suffering, we feel community, purpose and wholeness of being. Or for similar engagement with love's depth and mystery, meditate on Ernesto Cardenal's profound book *Love*.[30]

It is important to see the relationship between faith, hope, love and healing. The biblical stories of healing call for an attitude of expectant trust in God's power, that God will hear and answer the cry of the sufferer; they call for faith and courage to reach out toward God and ask for healing and wholeness. We should not pit faith healing against medical healing. We need not compartmentalize between the religious and the scientific, between natural and supernatural healing, between faith and pills. Rather, it is important to see the divine presence in healing whether it comes through the creative skills and abilities of the health professions, through the desperate prayer of the believer, or the community of faith practicing its religious heritage of exorcism, laying on of hands and anointing with oil. We open ourselves to the divine power and presence, pray humbly to God for healing for ourselves and others, rebuke the powers of evil that prey on human weakness, and be bearers of hope and loving care for each other, especially for those disabled who so much need the loving support of the community (see chap. 9).

In his book *Companions on the Inner Way*, Morton Kelsey ends with a chapter titled "The Mystery of Love." He quotes Carl Jung, saying that

---

[30]Ernesto Cardenal, *Love*, trans. Dinah Livingston (New York: Crossroad, 1981). This book, together with Ps 123:2; 125:1-2, was my daily meditation when I lay on my back and left side with right leg over left for ten days with severe lower back pain in 1981. On the tenth day my pain was gone.

our human capacity to love is much more important than our under-standings that arise from rational reflections. In Jung's own words, "I have again and again been faced with the mystery of love, and have never been able to explain what it is." Kelsey then directs his attention to the impor-tance of love in the helping professions:

> When all is said and done, the heart of all the helping professions is pro-viding an atmosphere of love in which people may be healed and then con-tinue to grow. I have no hard data, but I am convinced that behind almost all successful psychotherapy lies the hidden variable of concerned caring, of love. This probably as much as any other factor facilitates healing of mind, soul, emotions, body and society. However, as James Lynch points out so clearly in his book, *The Broken Heart*, love is difficult to define and does not fall into simple, objectively verifiable categories. Bruno Klopfer, the psy-chologist who established the use of the Rorschach test, once said to me that fifty percent of all psychotherapy is warm, accepting listening. This, he said, did not have to be confined to psychological professionals.[31]

Kelsey asks the reader to deal with anger and enmity also from the standpoint of love, for love is a power that can dissipate anger and turn enmity into friendship; it can free us from anger, hostility and the frustra-tions that arise from our human frailty and limitations of life. Jesus com-mands love for God, love for neighbor, love for one another and love for the enemy. This is Jesus Messiah's intended way for us to deal with hos-tilities, alienations and the frustrations that arise from our own human frailties and finitude, personally and corporately. Through our solidarity with and participation in the community (koinonia) of love and care, we find the way to live with and through these dilemmas of human suffering and human dignity in this world. Apostle Paul saw clearly this dilemma, believing in God's vindication of believers in the life to come:

> I want to know Christ and the power of his resurrection and the sharing of his sufferings by becoming like him in his death, if somehow I may attain the resurrection from the dead.
>
> Not that I have already obtained this or have already reached the goal; but I press on to make it my own, because Christ Jesus has made me his own. Beloved, I do not consider that I have made it my own; but this one

---

[31]Morton T. Kelsey, *Companions on the Inner Way: The Art of Spiritual Guidance* (New York: Crossroad, 1986), p. 197.

thing I do: forgetting what lies behind and straining forward to what lies ahead, I press on toward the goal for the prize of the heavenly call of God in Christ Jesus. . . .

But our citizenship is in heaven, and it is from there that we are expecting a Savior, the Lord Jesus Christ. He will transform the body of our humiliation that it may be conformed to the body of his glory, by the power that also enables him to make all things subject to himself. (Phil 3:10-14, 20-21)

4. Dying, we live.

This fourth paradox and mystery permeates New Testament thought. Jesus says in his teaching on discipleship,

If any want to become my followers, let them deny themselves and take up their cross and follow me. For those who want to save their life will lose it, and those who lose their life for my sake, and for the sake of the gospel, will save it. (Mk 8:34-35)

The same occurs in John's Gospel:

Very truly, I tell you, unless a grain of wheat falls into the earth and dies, it remains just a single grain; but if it dies, it bears much fruit. Those who love their life lose it, and those who hate [or give up] their life in this world will keep it for eternal life. (Jn 12:24-25)

Giving oneself in service to others, even unto death, enables finding true life and divine vindication (Mk 10:45; Phil 2:6-11). This is a central motif of the Gospels, in Jesus' death and resurrection. It provides the model for later catechetical teaching in the Epistles. For Paul baptism is death and resurrection (Rom 6:1-5). Baptism thus provides the model from 2 Corinthians 4:7-12, with verses 10-11 saying,

[We are] always carrying in the body the death of Jesus, so that the life of Jesus may also be made visible in our bodies. For while we live, we are always being given up to death for Jesus' sake, so that the life of Jesus may be made visible in our mortal flesh.

The principle applies even to one person giving his or her life in order that others might live: "So death is at work in us, but life in you" (v. 12), a point dramatically illustrated by missionary to India, Annie Funk, who gave up her life so another woman could survive in the sinking of the *Ti-*

tanic.[32] The Pauline pastoral epistles make the point a principle of faithfulness to gospel witness:

> Remember Jesus Christ, raised from the dead, a descendant of David—that is my gospel, for which I suffer hardship, even to the point of being chained like a criminal. But the word of God is not chained. Therefore I endure everything for the sake of the elect, so that they may also obtain the salvation that is in Christ Jesus, with eternal glory. The saying is sure:
> *If we have died with him, we will also live with him;*
> *if we endure, we will also reign with him.* (2 Tim 2:8-12, emphasis added)

The same writer earlier speaks of "the appearing of our Savior Christ Jesus, who abolished death and brought life and immortality to light through the gospel" (2 Tim 1:10). He anticipates his own dying and says assuredly,

> I have fought the good fight, I have finished the race, I have kept the faith. From now on there is reserved for me the crown of righteousness, which the Lord, the righteous judge, will give me on that day, and not only to me but also to all who have longed for his appearing. (2 Tim 4:7-8)

The Christian martyrs through the ages cry out with those in Revelation "How long, O Lord?" These martyrs throughout church history illustrate the paradox of "dying, we live." I recall with emotion the spontaneous lyric Ken Medema set to music to close a service at Eastern Mennonite University some years ago. While it is common to hear "Jesus died, that we might live" in much evangelical preaching and song, Medema sang it right, "Jesus died for us, so that we too might die, and live again."

As I write, my nephew-in-law is in his last hours of life, after battling a virulent cancer for a year. He said he is at peace and welcomes passing from this life to life with God in heaven. Heaven is where God is; we cannot fathom it. Dying for and in the Lord is the means by which we come to know joy, peace, and eternal hope (cf. 1 Pet 1:3-9).

Kenneth Bakken's convictions on the triune God's healing purpose identify what the church must do to reclaim its healing ministry, with the last my addition:

> First, she [the church] must clearly assert once again these basic assumptions:

---

[32]Sharon Yoder, *Annie Funk: Lived to Serve, Dared to Sacrifice*, illustrated by Jolynn Schmucker (Guy Mills, Penn.: Faith Builders Resource Group, 2008).

- The triune God is the source of all healing.

- God's will for us is *theosis*—transformation into the image of likeness of God.

- There is a spiritual, nonphysical reality, including good and evil forces.

- The cosmos is a dynamic creative energy, sanctified and sustained by God's loving.

- Body, mind, and spirit form an integrated whole.

- Healing occurs in many ways and is always more than a physical cure.

- Healing encompasses the gospel imperatives of justice, peacemaking, and service.[33]

- Caring for the dying is essential, as was the original vision of hospice.[34]

OUR CHRISTIAN HOPE

When Christ who is your [our] life is revealed,
then you [we] also will be revealed with him in glory. (Col 3:4)

Beloved, we are God's children now;
what we will be has not yet been revealed.
What we do know is this: when he is revealed,
we will be like him, for we will see him as he is. (1 Jn 3:2)

Do not let your hearts be troubled.
Believe in God, believe also in me.
In my Father's house there are many dwelling places.
If it were not so, would I have told you that I go to prepare a place for you?
And if I go and prepare a place for you,
I will come again and will take you to myself,
so that where I am, there you may be also. (Jn 14:1-3)

---

[33]Kenneth L. Bakken and Kathleen H. Hoffeller, *The Journey into God: Healing and the Christian Faith* (Minneapolis: Augsburg, 2000), pp. 5-6.

[34]Cicely Saunders, founder of the modern hospice ministry, reawakened the church to its historical ministry in caring for the sick, poor and dying (see chap. 8). Hospice, when done as Christian ministry is a valued alternative to what Allen Verhey calls "the medicalization of death" in "Still Dying Badly," *Christian Century*, November 1, 2011, pp. 22-27. On this point, see Amanda Bennett, "The Cost of Hope," *Newsweek*, June 4 & 11, 2012, pp. 52-55.

5

❖

The Church as Healing Community

O God, the source of all health; so fill my heart with faith in your love,
that with calm expectancy I may make room for your power to possess me,
and gracefully accept your healing, through Jesus Christ our Lord. Amen.

Book of Common Prayer

How does the church become a healing community? Two books with similar titles call the church to be God's healing people.[1] In 1993 my pastor, Duane Beck, and I led a seminar on healing at a churchwide conference. The many participants broke into small groups to share what healing ministries their congregations were engaged in during the last year. Their responses were:

- a twelve-step healing group in the congregation[2]
- a men's group studying and discussing healing
- a women's retreat on the healing dimensions of prayer
- a Sunday morning sermon series on healing
- mediation efforts focused on healing
- Stephen Ministries

---

[1]Frank Bateman Stanger, *God's Healing Community* (Wilmore, Ky.: Francis Asbury, 1985), and Karin Granberg-Michaelson, *Healing Community* (Geneva: WCC Publications, 1991). The latter is more broadly based in thought, and, like the first, is directed to the church. Another helpful contribution is Al Dueck, "The Church as a Healing Community," *Builder* 41 (1991): 2-8.

[2]James Douglas Nelson, *Awakening: Restoring Health Through the Spiritual Principles of Shalom, Jesus and the Twelve Step Recovery Program* (Blue Ridge Summit, Penn.: TAB Books, 1989).

- Sunday evening anointing service
- anointing the sick upon personal request

Since the mid-eighties my home church, Belmont Mennonite, has had at the end of the service, about every sixth Sunday, prayers for healing for those coming forward. Since healing and wholeness are intrinsic to the gospel, we must reassess our notions about health care (see part 3). What will it take to recapture the fundamental vision that health care is, first and foremost, a religious privilege?

Think about this for a moment. Who gives life and health? Do nations bestow life and health? Does the medical profession bestow life and health? Since God is the giver of life and the one who bestows health, enabling healing as a creative gift, then all health care services can be viewed as ministry to some degree. Stanley Hauerwas pinpoints the issue by asking why we put more faith in pills than we do in God for healing. He regards this to be a theodicy issue and devotes most of his book to this topic! As he puts it:

> Sickness challenges our most cherished presumption that we are or at least can be in control of our existence. Sickness creates the problem of "anthropodicy" because it challenges our most precious and profound belief that humanity has in fact become god. Against the backdrop of such a belief, we conclude that sickness should not exist.
>
> In such a context, medicine becomes the mirror image of theoretical theodicies sponsored by the Enlightenment because it attempts to save our profoundest hopes that sickness should and can be eliminated. We must assume a causal order so that this new emperor can be assured of success. We do not need a community capable of caring for the ill; all we need is an instrumental rationality made powerful by technological sophistication.[3]

For perspective to resolve this dilemma that modern medicine creates for us—resulting in double-talk: lip service to God as healer but practical obeisance to medicine as healer—we need to read again Sirach 38:1-15 to understand that the skills of the physicians, pharmacists and other health

---

[3]Stanley Hauerwas, *Naming the Silences: God, Medicine, and the Problem of Suffering* (Grand Rapids: Eerdmans, 1990), p. 62. Hauerwas then notes that earlier it was assumed physicians should not *act* unless such was necessary; now physicians assume their first responsibility is to *act*. Thus, "physicians lose their freedom to care for the sick because they are not judged by the predictability of their performance" (pp. 63-64).

care professionals function to support God's healing of our sicknesses, even when "cures" are not possible. The physician *assists* God in bestowing health. Sickness is not God's absence. Medical cures rooted in scientific knowledge do not negate God as healer who gives wholeness and well-being. Rooted in human nature in creation and manifest in Jesus' gift of salvation, healing is God's gift through creation and grace. This means that doctors, nurses, and pharmacists are synergistic to God's work of healing. Health care personnel are thus called to be proactive partners in God's gift of healing.

CULTURAL FACTORS AND BIBLICAL PERSPECTIVES

Two stories, in counterpoint, exemplify differing attitudes toward illness and healing. In the fall of 1987 at Anabaptist Mennonite Biblical Seminary, a new Nigerian student met me in the hall and asked how I was—his culture's customary greeting. I said I was fine. But he then inquired of my family. I told him that Mary, my wife, was recovering slowly from a broken leg. He immediately expressed concern and then inquired whether he and his wife could visit Mary to pray with her. He said he didn't know how it is in American culture, but he is concerned about Mary's leg because one of his Nigerian friends had the bad experience of having his wife become ill while they were in America, and no one visited her. In Nigeria, he said, it is very important for a sick person to be visited by many friends. If not, the person will not get well. Indeed, Obed and Phena came and visited Mary the next day, and prayed for her healing.[4]

A few days later I told this story to two seminary students in the coffee lounge. One student's immediate response was that of his own contrasting family culture. He said his father would never admit to being ill; he never would miss work even though when sick. If anyone else in the family, mother or children, did admit to being ill, it was expected they would withdraw, likely go to their rooms and stay there for most of the day (or days) until they got well. In this scenario, sickness isolates one from community!

---

[4]The importance of pastoral visitation of the sick is high on the expected duties of a pastor. For a Lutheran pastor's analysis of the importance of visiting the sick, drawing on the early and later church fathers, see Philip H. Pfatteicher, "Some Early and Later Fathers on the Visitation of the Sick," *Pro Ecclesia* 19, no. 2 (2010): 207-22. The article richly blends biblical and historical convictions, including present practice.

These stories illustrate contrasting practices regarding sickness and healing. We might ask, What are the strengths and weaknesses of both models? And in which society would we like to be when we are sick or disabled?

What are some of the biblical practices and images for healing? Certain biblical stories readily come into focus: in the Old Testament the story of the Syrian army captain Naaman coming to Israel's prophet Elisha shines. Naaman finds healing through a humble trustful act—with urging from his servants when he is in a huff by such a ridiculous command—of dipping seven times in the muddy Jordan River (2 Kings 5:1-19).[5] Another, in the New Testament, tells of a paralytic carried by four friends onto a housetop and let down through the roof. Jesus heals by command, "Stand up and take your mat and walk," together with implied forgiveness of sins (Mk 2:1-12; contrast here Jn 9:1-2).[6] These are strong, powerful images. We use these stories most frequently to address the issue of faith. But another crucial point must be made; in both cases the sick person's help came through friends.

In the first story this is touching because it is a young captive maiden girl from Israel that initiates reaching out on behalf of the Syrian captain, with Syria sometimes in enemy relation to Israel. The story shows the struggle of the captain with feelings of foolishness and vulnerability that accompany such a risky endeavor. The second story has its own arresting twist; the friends of the paralytic are so confident of Jesus' power to heal that they go to great lengths to get the paralytic to Jesus.

These stories illustrate points applicable to us: courage to reach out for help, helpers who risk themselves to find resources for healing, and expression of faith in a public communal context. In Naaman's story national and personal hostilities are transcended for healing to occur. Also we hear the sufferer's cry for help and willingness to be vulnerable.

---

[5]For extended exposition of this healing, see Frederick Gaiser, *Healing in the Bible: Theological Insight for Christian Ministry* (Grand Rapids: Eerdmans, 2010), pp. 63-73.

[6]See Gaiser also for good treatment of this healing under the title "Your Sins Are Forgiven . . . Stand Up and Walk," pp. 191-206. The role of friends in this story is especially striking, as well as Jesus' word of forgiveness to the sick man, which prompts the religious leaders to judge Jesus as a blasphemer, since only God can forgive sins (see Jn 5:1-18 for a similar story and conclusion by Jewish leaders who then start to persecute Jesus, v. 16). Gaiser does not include John 5 in his selection; it is similar in effect to Mark 2.

BIBLICAL PRACTICES

In Christian teaching and practice certain symbolic practices and images carry healing power. I mention seven healing images/rituals (some of these are sacraments in the Roman Catholic Church).[7]

1. Baptism: Cross and resurrection. Sacramental symbols of power for healing, baptism, cross, and resurrection belong together in light of the early church's catechetic practices of preparing candidates for baptism. The church engaged the candidate for baptism in extended teaching on new life in Christ together with prayers to expel evil spirits. After a year or more (sometimes three) this culminated in baptism, the final exorcism. In baptism we die to the old life and are raised into new life (Rom 6:1-4; Col 3:1-3). This catechetical process climaxing in baptism initiates the believer into Christ-directed living, in which catechumens change emperors to rule their lives: Jesus Christ, not Satan; the Christian community, not the political emperor.

Though the cross was not used publicly as a symbol of salvation in the second to third centuries, Paul sums up the gospel as preaching Christ crucified, with the cross central to the gospel narrative (1 Cor 1:18–2:4; Gal 6:14). Through the cross and resurrection Jesus sets us free from bondage to the evil one and gives us the authority to set others free in his name. Prayer for spiritual freedom (i.e., deliverance from evil powers) is usually in the form of a command "in the name of Jesus" (Acts 3–4). This prayer may be spoken with reverence and authority,

> Lord Jesus, we rejoice in your victory over Satan and sin.
> We rejoice that you share your victory with us.
> Lord, in your name and with your authority, I bind every evil spirit.

When we bind Satan in the name of Jesus, his power is restrained. He is bound. The celebrant pronounces freedom in the name of Jesus: In the name of Jesus I break free from bondage to . . . (e.g., drugs, pornography, harbored hatred, etc.). The celebrant then leads the congregation in prayers of thanks and praise. "Lord, we bless you that you have overcome the

---

[7]Francis MacNutt discusses seven sacraments (differing from mine). He says that in the practice of six of them he witnessed healings (*Healing* [Notre Dame, Ind.: Ave Maria Press, 1999], pp. 219-36). Baptism, Lord's Supper and anointing with oil occur in both his and my seven. My "foot-washing" combined with "Lord's Supper" are similar to his fifth, "confession of sins" and forgiveness, which, he says, is now called "reconciliation."

world; we praise you, Lord, because you have set us free."[8]

Taking authority against evil spirits is not to be used for most sickness, but only for those illnesses intertwined with addictive patterns of behavior in which the person is helpless under the grip of demonic powers (occasioned sometimes by participation in the occult, inviting demons into one's life or pledge of allegiance to Satan). Although there are numerous ways in which God's liberating power is appropriated for the benefit of such a person's healing (Ps 3 and Ps 91 have been used historically for this purpose), it is important that such be done within a community (never alone, except in follow-up for spiritual nurture). A liturgical form for such encounter is helpful, assuming all those participating mean the words they say.

The cross reconciles alienated peoples and turns hostilities into a bond of peace. Consider again the healing potential of the cross, whether we see it in the church behind the pulpit, on the Communion table or worn on a person's necklace. The cross is God's nonretaliatory weapon of victory and triumph over evil; it is Christ's provision for our healing and shalom.[9] The cross as source of healing is a mysterious paradox—in how Jesus' suffering, even as a criminal, heals us, "upon him was the punishment that made us whole [*shalom*]" (NRSV), Isaiah puts in poetic parallel healing and wholeness. Isaiah 53:5 says it memorably: "by his wounds we are healed [*rapha*]" (NIV, TNIV, NET and 1 Peter 2:24); "with his stripes we are healed" [KJV; cf. REB].[10] Indeed, in our baptisms we are coburied into Christ with the promise that we are thereby also coraised into Christ (Rom 6:1-14; Phil 2:5-11; 3:7-12; Col 3:1-4).

---

[8]My revision of similar statements from Jim McManus, *The Healing Power of the Sacraments* (Notre Dame, Ind.: Ave Maria Press, 1984), pp. 94-95. For fuller treatment of deliverance practice see my (Swartley) articles in *Even the Demons Submit: Continuing the Ministry of Jesus*, ed. Loren Johns and James Krabill (Scottdale, Penn.: Herald Press, 2007), pp. 24-40, 108-15, 177, 181-99; *Transforming the Powers: Peace, Justice, and the Domination System*, ed. Ray Gingerich and Ted Grimsrud (Minneapolis, Fortress, 2006), pp. 96-112, 143-56; *Jesus Matters*, ed. James Krabill and David W. Shenk (Scottdale, Penn.: Herald Press, 2009), pp. 89-103. For use of the Eucharist as a sacramental ritual for deliverance, see Tilda Norberg, *Consenting to Grace: An Introduction to Gestalt Pastoral Care* (New York: Penn House, 2006), pp. 266-69, and deliverance procedure without the Eucharist (ibid., pp. 263-65, 269-70).
[9]Erland Waltner, "Shalom and Wholeness," *Brethren Life and Thought* 29 (1984): 147-49.
[10]For extended discussion of these verses in relation to atonement, see Darrin Snyder Belousek, *Atonement, Justice, and Peace: The Message of the Cross and the Mission of the Church* (Grand Rapids: Eerdmans, 2012), pp. 232-34, 237, 243.

Through the cross we are reconciled to others, even to our enemies. As the classic reconciliation text in 2 Corinthians 5:17-20 says, reconciliation is God's work and also our task. In chiasm, we observe the importance of God's initiative (the central D unit):

A In Christ, all is *new creation* (old passed away; all become new)
　B All this is from God, who reconciled us to himself through Christ,
　　C and has given us the ministry of reconciliation;
　　　D that is, in Christ God was reconciling the world to himself,
　　　　not counting their trespasses against them, and
　　C' entrusting the message of reconciliation to us.
　　　So we are ambassadors for Christ,
　　　since God is making his appeal through us;
　B' we entreat you on behalf of Christ, be reconciled to God.
A' that we might become the righteousness of God.[11]

Healing through reconciliation is *God's* gift (D); second, it is *our* task (C and C'). This is the archetypal pattern of the church's healing ministry. Reconciliation may occur in any and all of these images and practices.

2. *The Lord's Supper/Eucharist and the love feast, with foot washing.* In Virginia some years ago while attending a conference on Anabaptism I participated in a Church of the Brethren love feast. This, with the Communion, was truly a high point. It enacted the healing power of the community. It oriented our common life to Jesus.

The meal is a fellowship meal, a distinctive type of fellowship (koinonia), a fellowship bound to the life and death of Jesus Christ. I see two streams of emphasis in the Lord's Supper that contribute significantly to the healing and health of the congregation. The one is common fellowship. Combining the foot washing, love feast and Communion draws us in spirit into the heart of caring love. We are in the presence of the holy, a common holy, in which the ordinary elements of food, water, cup and bread bond the new community, the new creation begun by Jesus. Healing prayer may be combined also with this service.

Participating in the sacred meal with demeaning attitudes toward one another exacerbates our brokenness and illness. In 1 Corinthians 11:27-32

---

[11]See the similar chiasm in V. George Shillington's *2 Corinthians*, Believers Church Bible Commentary (Scottdale, Penn.: Herald Press, 1999), p. 127. Shillington has excellent discussion of this passage, setting it within the wider letter context.

Paul explicitly links unworthy participation in the Eucharist to the moral failure and health of people in the community. Paul's judgment of the Corinthians' Lord's Supper practice lay in their alienating division between the rich and the poor. The rich apparently came first and ate most of the choice food. When the poor who worked late arrived, there was little food left. The issue is not only that some were well-filled and some remained hungry, but that the difference underscored sharply the socio-economic disparity within the community. Paul dares to say that this situation is the cause of illness, sickness and even death among some of the members. May such favoritism and injustice not be in our Communion or, perhaps more relevant, in our potluck meals.

A second dimension of healing is the holiness of the Lord's Supper. The Lord's Supper commemorates the death of Jesus, God's resurrection victory and the future final triumph of God's people. It puts believers in touch with the depth reality of faith and the interplay between that faith and living it in our religious practices. God's *presence* is mediated into our human situation. That presence is power, a power that can heal the sick, whether it is physical, emotional or spiritual sickness.

On one of my sabbaticals I attended an Episcopal church, where I found healing in the Eucharist with these words as we took the Communion emblems: "The broken body and shed blood of the Lord Jesus Christ keep you in body, soul, and spirit until the day of his coming."

In Roman Catholic churches, the Eucharist liturgy sometimes is linked to healing, as in this post-Communion prayer:

> Lord, through this sacrament may we rejoice in your healing power and experience your love in mind and body. Lord, our God, renew us by these mysteries. May they heal us now and bring us to eternal salvation.[12]

By attending to the healing power of these symbols and the dynamics of the divine-human dimension at work and between humans, we worthily celebrate the Lord's Supper and experience God's healing presence within the fellowship of believers.

3. *Laying on of hands and anointing with oil.* Laying on of hands and anointing with oil symbolize our recognition of God's divine power needed for our healing; oil is a natural healing ingredient, long recog-

---

[12]McManus, *Healing Power of the Sacraments*, pp. 78-79.

nized as a healing balm. In the early church these two specific practices emerged as expressions of the church's empowerment to heal (Jas 5:13-18). James connects anointing with oil to confession of sins (v. 16). Opportunity for confession witnesses to the wholeness of the person, the relation of the spiritual to the physical. Anointing with oil should not be reserved for only extreme illness or last rites. Laying on of hands and anointing with oil powerfully testify to the humble dependence of the community on God. It witnesses to the support of brothers and sisters as they gather around the one to be healed. It vulnerably opens each person to the transcendent presence and power of God. What a treasure for churches to give opportunity for confession of sins and anoint with oil for healing.

As Dean Miller of the Church of the Brethren says, "Healing will occur in a congregation where accepting, caring, forgiving, and loving people unite in prayer and demonstrate support to those who come seeking to be anointed."[13]

Several key questions arise in relation to this practice:

- Who takes the initiative? Must the sick person ask for anointing? While the sick person might desire the anointing, the initiative for it may come from the sick person, a family member, the pastor or someone else in the congregation. Discernment and a common mind and spirit are important. The Church of the Brethren points the way, for its practice of anointing with oil is expected as the church's gift in healing ministry.

- What about anointing nonmembers, even non-Christians? We have no clear word from Scripture on this, but the Gospel narratives of healing indicate that healing is part of the proclamation of the kingdom gospel. In these cases the healing ministry functions as invitational to enter the kingdom, to become part of the body. In mission ministries in areas new to the gospel, healing often precedes and leads to belief.

- Must confession of sin be part of a healing ritual? We need not be legalistic on this. But if we are knowingly hiding sin, forget anointing. Sin should be dealt with first. I like the way Phyllis Carter put it in a sermon at AMBS from the Church of the Brethren practice: "Is there any sin which you know that would keep this prayer from being effectual?" The

[13]Dean M. Miller, "Anointing: An Ancient Rite in New Settings," *Messenger*, June 1987, pp. 26-27.

gospel relates forgiveness of sin and healing. James 5:16 links confession and healing.

4. Word. The image of spoken word, caring word, compassionate word is central to Scripture. We live in a world of many competing demands on our time. It is easy to overlook the importance of speaking a caring word to someone who suffers, who is ill and lonely in their illness. This is why my Nigerian friend believes it important to visit the sick. The visit brings presence and word to counter loneliness, alienation and low self-worth because of one's sickness or disability.

The significance of *word* for healing flows in two directions. First, there is the need for the compassionate word to be spoken to the one who is ill. But there is also the need for the word of petition and cry for help from the one who is ill. Jeremiah's outcry for healing help is pointed and potent:

Heal me, O LORD, and I shall be healed;
  save me, and I shall be saved;
  for you are my praise. (Jer 17:14)

The healing power of *word* is evident in the resurgence of biblical story-telling. The learning and telling of biblical stories, especially healing stories, can transform both the teller and the hearer. Telling Bible stories to the disabled, or reciting Scripture together, renews the spirit and generates healing power for the mind and body; it opens up the deeper levels of feeling, providing an entree into the inner depths of the hurting, aching self.

Related to the image of word is the *renewing of the mind*, of which Scripture speaks several times (Rom 12:2; Eph 4:23). The texts that speak specifically of renewing of the mind are those in which a change from old life to new life is envisioned. Renewing the mind means renouncing former patterns of behavior and opening oneself to the newness and transforming power of the gospel.

5. The heart. In *Healing the Heart*, Joseph Grassi shows how central heart language is to the biblical text. The word is used over 850 times in the Old Testament (see Ps 28:7 as example, there used twice) and 150 in the New.[14] In modern speech, however, the word *heart* has been relegated

[14]Joseph Grassi, *Healing the Heart: The Transformational Power of Biblical Heart Imagery* (New York: Paulist Press, 1987), p. 20. Grassi says the Oxford Dictionary of the English Language

to Valentine's Day and medical cardiology departments, including heart transplants. Unlike biblical language, we seldom use the word *heart* to describe our feelings, will, desires, thoughts, remembering, relationships and unity. As Grassi points out, "heart language is becoming more and more suppressed."[15] This contributes to increasing stress in our modern technological world.

Studies have demonstrated the connection between stress and heart illnesses. Suppression of heart language results in suppression and constriction of the heart itself. Excessive concentration on informational computer-type language means that we effectively tell the heart to hold back. This most likely played a role in my own heart attack, since then I was working overtime at the computer (see the introduction).

By way of contrast, biblical heart language conveys emotion. The Old Testament uses the emphatic personal pronoun *I* only six or seven times. Feelings are expressed with heart language: my heart is heavy, joyful, warm, sad, broken and so forth. *Heart* designates the totality of the human person, which some medical personnel and practices are now recovering. Biblical heart language helps us to recover this holistic view, as this prayer, my brother's in dealing with his heart illness, voices:

> In this time of health needs, Jesus, touch my emotions,
> lest through illness I die and return to dust.
> When You see me trembling bring to me the Holy Spirit.
> the Presence hovering over my soul, body, and spirit.
> And once more let me experience joy overflowing
> like waters bursting from the ever-flowing stream.[16]

6. Feasts and celebrations. Over the years I have become increasingly surprised by the significance of feasts, eating and celebrations in Scripture. In the Old Testament each family participated in three major feasts annually, often involving a one- to three-day journey, to and fro. These feasts heightened the community's sense of belonging to God: time and land

---

has fifty-six categories of meaning for *heart*. Only four refer to the physical heart. The current dominant use of heart language pertains to cardiology. I know; it's true for me.

[15]Ibid. Flora Slosson Wuellner's *Heart of Healing, Heart of Light: Encountering God Who Shares and Heals Our Pain* (Nashville: Upper Room Books, 1992) is a good remedy for this morass.

[16]Henry Swartley, "Hold Me, Lord!" in *Living on the Fault Line: Portrait and Journals of a Church Planter Pastor*, ed. Willard Swartley (Nappanee, Ind.: Evangel Press, 1992), adapted from vv. 2-3, p. 30 (entry on March 10, 1987).

were viewed as God's gifts. They celebrated God's ownership in the feasts.

The first and foundational feast was Passover, a celebration of the Lord's deliverance from death. As the exodus story narrates God's deliverance and the people's praise, the Lord promises health protection as bonus to their salvation: "I will not bring upon you any of the diseases that I brought upon the Egyptians; for I am the LORD who heals you" (Ex 15:26). They understood their covenant community was bonded to God as their redeemer, defender and healer of infirmities.

Israel also celebrated the feast of the firstfruits and the feast of tabernacles, the latter a time of retreat into the wilderness and living in tents. The Passover and tabernacles feasts were each full-week affairs. These celebrations functioned as healing balm for the soul, providing and enhancing community life. They brought moments of solemn worship, but also much joy, vitality and laughter.

Similarly, the early church followed Jesus' celebrative table fellowship practices by including Jews and Gentiles around the same table, participating as the body of Christ in the healing power of the Eucharist. One of the emphases in studies on the historical Jesus is his commensality: table fellowship with people from all walks of life.

7. *The kiss of peace* or *passing of peace*. In connection with our celebrations of the Lord's Supper and other special events in the life of God's people, the kiss of peace (or embrace) can be a significant practice, with healing effect. In our culture and world where closeness and touch have been virtually eliminated or have been prostituted in the erotic dimensions of our modern Hollywood and TV culture, the restoration of this act within the context of worship can be a powerful way to break down alienating barriers that reinforce illness and the causes that underlie illness. Granted, we must consider also the cultural hazards in using this symbol for healing in light of the meanings that our culture has put on it. I suggest we teach more about the symbol and its use in our congregations. Perhaps "passing the peace" is our best alternative. How do we release the power of this symbol for those with disabilities that make it difficult to embrace, kiss or pass the peace? Are these persons slighted in giving and receiving emotional warmth?

These seven images or practices aid the Christian church's healing ministry. If you use this book in a class for study, discuss the following: to what extent does *our* church engage in these practices? What role do these practices or images have in our congregation or in our personal lives? Do we pray for the health of our congregation and community?

CONCLUSION

Karin Granberg-Michaelson calls churches to examine our healing commitments:

- Are we and our churches healing communities?
- Are we really engaging ourselves in God's controversy with those who spread sickness around?
- Are we enabling our sick people and societies to diagnose their true sickness and find resources for healing?
- Are we prepared to place ourselves beside the sick, the deprived, the oppressed with the healing power of God?
- Are we ready to join our Lord in his self-giving struggle with evil even to the cross in order that healing, reconciliation and wholeness may become manifest in a world which is sick to death?[17]

In the Lord's Prayer (Mt 6:9-13) we pray for God's healing reign to come to earth:

Our Father in heaven,
   hallowed be your name.
   Your kingdom come.
   Your will be done,
      on earth as it is in heaven.

---

[17]Karin Granberg-Michaelson, *Healing Community* (Geneva: WCC Publications, 1991), p. 14.

PART TWO

Health Care

Biblical, Moral and
Theological Perspectives

6

❖

Health and Health Care in
Biblical-Theological Perspective

Happy are those whose help is the God of Jacob,
whose hope is in the LORD their God, . . .
who executes justice for the oppressed;
who gives food to the hungry.

The LORD sets the prisoners free;
the LORD opens the eyes of the blind.
The LORD lifts up those who are bowed down;
the LORD loves the righteous.
The LORD watches over the strangers;
he upholds the orphan and the widow.

Psalm 146:5-9

Let justice roll down like waters,
and righteousness like an ever flowing stream.

Amos 5:24

You shall love your neighbor as yourself.

Leviticus 19:18; Luke 10:27

What guides our understanding of health and our views on health care reform? Do we derive our views of health from a naturalist perspective or a biblical-theological perspective? Is health care primarily a medical or economic-political issue? Or is it first and foremost a moral matter rooted in Scripture and theological reflection? The dual goal of this chapter is to help us better understand what we mean by *health* and explain why health care is a moral priority.

These cited biblical verses reveal God's will for humans: shalom for one's self and one's neighbor, including health; justice for oneself and for all in the community, especially the poor; and help for the marginalized and the "other." In Luke 10:25-37 the neighbor is a Samaritan, the people despised by the Jews, indeed, the enemy. These Scriptures ask us to rethink health and the purposes of health care. It's a matter of shalom and justice for all, with hospitality to the poor and marginalized. The Samaritan's health care for the wounded Jew turns tables upside down in regard to dominant moral expectations. It is not the priest or Levite but the hated Samaritan whom we call good who provides the needed health care and restores the wounded to health. What can we learn from this story? Who is our neighbor in need of health care and restored health?

Allen Ginsberg reflects on the tragedy in Tucson, Arizona (January 8, 2011), from the standpoint of transcending divisions in our country: a Republican Catholic judge goes with his Jewish friend to hear Democratic Representative Gabrielle Giffords address and listen to people's political concerns on Safeway's parking lot—her "Congress on the Corner." When Giffords was shot in the head, a Latino intern promptly provides first aid to stop her bleeding, likely saving her life. The chief hospital surgeon for Rep. Giffords is Korean American. The U.S. President, who comes to share and represent the nation's grief and extend sympathy, is African American. These responses show how a tragic crisis grips the heart and brings people together across party, racial and ethnic lines.

Are our basic Christian understandings of health and convictions about health care based on the moral vision of biblical teaching?

1. What is a tenable view of health, based in Scripture and Christian theology?

2. Is access to health care for all citizens and residents in the United States a moral issue? Or put differently, do all people have a moral right to health care access?

3. Should we consider health and health care simply as a "human rights" matter or is there something specifically Christian in our concern?

4. Is health care only a justice issue? Is it part of Christian *mission* as well?

Five Biblical Themes and Early Christian Practices

Five biblical themes and early Christian practices speak to our understanding of health and why universal health care access is important:

1. In Scripture, shalom (well-being) is God's will and desire for all people. *Shalom*, the Hebrew word for "peace" (used around 250 times in the Old Testament) has many dimensions of meaning: wholeness, well-being, peace, salvation and justice. Shalom occurs often in inquiring about one's welfare (Gen 29:6; 37:14; 43:27; Ex 18:7; 1 Sam 10:4; 17:18, 22; 25:5; 30:21). Inquiry about a person's "welfare includes everything necessary to healthful living: good health, a sense of well-being, good fortune, the cohesiveness of the community, relationship to relatives and their state of being, and anything else deemed necessary for everything to be in order."[1] English versions on occasion translate *shalom* as prosperity (Ps 37:11; Is 54:13). Shalom also has moral connotations: it is the opposite of deceit (Ps 34:13-14; Jer 8:22–9:6); it requires truth and transparency in relationships.

Shalom assumes relationship with God and meaningful relationships with fellow humans. Cheating others, hurting others in any way, violating covenants and living selfishly deprive the community of shalom, health in its fullness. Such actions impede shalom health. Similarly, when some people are deprived of access to health care, shalom is also compromised. When a health care system excludes the most vulnerable citizens from basic, nonemergency health care coverage, it denies shalom to those people. Such exclusion obstructs God's gift of shalom for humans. For further discussion of shalom and its significance for health care, see chapter eleven.

---

[1] Claus Westermann, "Peace [*Shalom*] in the Old Testament," in *The Meaning of Peace*, ed. Perry B. Yoder and Willard M. Swartley (Elkhart, Ind.: Institute of Mennonite Studies, 2001), p. 49.

It is essential, however, to affirm that *health* as such is not the chief goal and purpose of life. Health or health care dare not become our idol. While we value health and laud universal health care access, we must recognize also that health is a gift, not something money can buy.[2] Shalom means more than good health, and it can be experienced when one is sick or disabled. Marva Dawn persuasively makes this point and exemplifies it in her own experience. She contributes shalom to others through her gift of writing, even though she lives with numerous health limitations.[3]

Shalom and *health* cannot be equated; shalom cannot be reduced to health. Though one's shalom may be threatened by failed health or disability, people with poor health or disability can also experience and testify to God's shalom in their lives. Health is not the make-all or end-all of life lived as God desires. As Mary McDonough says in her provocative book *Can a Health Care Market Be Moral?* the definition of health endorsed by the World Health Organization (WHO) is too broad: "Health is a state of complete physical, mental, and social well-being and not merely the absence of disease or infirmity."[4] To the extent this definition embraces a holistic view of wellness, it is on target. But, negatively, it tends to make *health* the chief goal of life. Rather, "health is an essential part of life but not the goal of life."[5] Health serves a larger vision and goal for life. To focus on the body and its health can become idolatry in our present body-health culture.[6] The meaning and fulfillment "of life are found [rather] in human *relationships*, and qualities of justice, respect, concern, compassion, and support that surround" those relationships and qualities.[7] All these factors contribute to personal and corporate shalom.

Another critique of the WHO definition of health lies in its failure to recognize that some decisions, vocations and actions are more important than health. If that were not so, Jewish and Christian history would have no martyrs. Fewer people would heed the call to risk-taking missionary

---

[2]See Rodney Clapp, "Health Money Can't Buy," *Christian Century*, September 22, 2009, p. 45.

[3]Marva J. Dawn, *Being Well When We're Ill: Wholeness and Hope in Spite of Infirmity* (Minneapolis: Augsburg, 2008).

[4]Mary McDonough, *Can a Health Care Market Be Moral? A Catholic Vision* (Washington, D.C.: Georgetown University Press, 2007), pp. 164-65.

[5]Ibid., p. 213.

[6]This is one of the cautions in the instructive book *Christian Faith, Health, and Medical Practice*, ed. Hessel Bouma III et al. (Grand Rapids: Eerdmans, 1989), pp. 4-5.

[7]Richard McCormick, cited in McDonough, *Can a Health Care Market Be Moral?* p. 211.

work. Some pastors would immediately resign. Competitive sports, with all its hazards to health, would fall under strong cultural critique. In an insightful article Neil Messer takes up this critique of WHO's definition of health and rightly critiques it on the basis of failing to recognize that the Christian vision for life is larger than health.[8] However, part of his critique seems flawed in that he begins by labeling the WHO definition as a "theory of everything."[9] Rather, its weakness is its failure to see that health is not *everything*, a point he makes as his essay progresses. He rightly affirms Karl Barth's discussion of health under the rubric "Freedom to Live," with definition of health as "strength for human life."[10] "Freedom to live" means freedom to live for God and for others, which may entail risk-taking actions to one's health (witness Jesus!). As Messer contends, the WHO definition may appeal to a "naturalist" view of health, but it fails to place health within the larger goal of living for God and others, even at the peril of one's health. Jesus' own life and dying is the prime example (cf. the "Servant of the Lord" description in Is 53:2-6). Paul's "thorn in the flesh" (2 Cor 12:7) also demonstrates that Paul, the risk-taking apostle, sacrifices health for his mission commitment (2 Cor 11:23-32). Paul's theology contends that God's power is manifest in our human weakness. Our ultimate goal in life is to be like Jesus Christ and, as chapter nine narrates, that goal is often achieved by the disabled.[11]

Dying and death must also be included in our vision of shalom. Scripture calls us to put our trust in the Lord. Trusting the Lord for day-to-day guidance and empowerment brings wholeness of mind and body. Current literature emphasizes this, stressing the mind and body connection. The insight is ancient, as Proverbs tells us:

> Trust in the LORD with all your heart,
>   and do not rely on your own insight.
> In all your ways acknowledge him,

---

[8]Neil Messer, "Toward a Theological Understanding of Health and Disease," *Journal of the Society of Christian Ethics* 31, no. 1 (2011): 161-78.

[9]Ibid., pp. 162-64.

[10]Ibid., pp. 166-71.

[11]Messer refers to the example of "Dorothy," an assistant Sunday school teacher with Down Syndrome, described by Stanley Hauerwas and William H. Willimon in *Resident Aliens* as an exemplary saint, for whose funeral in her local Methodist church the whole congregation came ("Toward a Theological Understanding of Health and Disease," p. 172)

and he will make straight your paths.
Do not be wise in your own eyes;
     fear the LORD, and turn away from evil.
It will be a healing for your flesh
     and a refreshment for your body. (Prov 3:5-8)

Healing and refreshment of the body are the *fruit* of trusting in the Lord, which require fearing the Lord and turning away from evil. But we cannot deduce from this that all sickness is the result of sin or failure to trust the Lord. Job sets us straight on this point, as does Jesus in John 9:1-2, in refusing his disciples' assumption that the man was born blind because either he or his parents had sinned. Rowan Williams aptly says, "Christians have every reason to say no to any system . . . that uses suffering to prove things: to prove the sufferer's guilt as a sinner being punished, or to prove the sufferer's innocence as a martyr." Rather, the blind man's condition opens up a space "where communication from God occurs."[12]

When we confess God or Jesus as healer we raise a practical issue for us who enjoy the benefits of modern medicine. If faithful Israel trusted in God as healer and also affirmed use of medical and pharmaceutical resources, then we may blend the two also, or better, recognize that the two blend intrinsically in God's healing design (see Sir 38:1-4, 6-10, 12-15). Luke the physician exemplifies this blend in his Gospel. As a physician, according to early church tradition, he accentuates Jesus' healing ministry. Luke sums up Jesus' ministry with two major motifs: Jesus' proclamation of the peace gospel, and his healing ministry, including exorcisms (Acts 10:36-38). These are the hallmarks of Jesus' identity.

From my own hospital experiences I know the importance of this blend for healing, a combination of medical expertise and a perseverant praying, loving and caring community. With only one of these, I would likely not be living now to write this book. Recognizing the intertwining of these two contributions to healing and health gives us a grateful spirit for whatever health we have, even when compromised.

The Lord (God, Jesus, Spirit) is ultimately the one who heals ("I am the LORD who heals you," Ex 15:26). Medical knowledge and skill with its ability to cure, and the praying, caring church contribute to God's healing

---

[12]Rowan Williams, *Writing in the Dust: Reflections on 11th September and Its Aftermath* (London: Hodder & Stoughton, 2002), pp. 75-76.

work. These three working together enable shalom personally and communally. Given this perspective we can avoid loading onto the medical profession unlimited expectations, playing God and ending up with a health care system that is unsustainable, due to rampant individualism and an ever-increasing sense of entitlement to all technologies and heroic measures to save one's life. In contrast to this pervasive assumption of health insurance entitlement, the Amish emphasize *Gelassenheit*, a yielding to God's and their community's care for them, come what may.

In a capitalist and individualist society, with a market-driven health care system and ever-developing costly technology, health care for all becomes increasingly unsustainable.[13] The health care crisis is symptomatic. It is indicative of how deeply immersed and addicted our culture has become to greediness. Even in hospice, some for-profit organizations market service, for a profit, to the terminally ill. Until we begin to face our addictions to money and "prosperity," we will remain as an oppressive society, especially to the sick and destitute.

Some limits are required to what we expect and seek to do in medical care, especially its technology. Downing calls this system "biomedicine," a term that combines modern medical research and practice with technology and a profit motive driving it. We indeed face the risk of idolizing health and health care entitlements, with God's and the church's role in health care forgotten (see the Hauerwas quote at the beginning of chap. 5). Downing, a medical doctor practicing in Kenya, acknowledges the good of biomedicine, able often to cure and heal. But its political power is a prime force driving Western global imperialism in the twenty-first century. He includes it in the "principalities and powers" of our time, clouding our vision of God's reign and the priority of the gospel.[14]

---

[13]See the good discussion of this problem by Maggie Mahar, *Money-Driven Medicine: The Real Reason Health Care Costs So Much* (New York: Harper Collins, 2005).

[14]Raymond Downing, *Death and Life in America: Biblical Healing and Biomedicine* (Scottdale, Penn.: Herald Press, 2008), pp. 25-84, esp. pp. 43-45, 68-69. Downing is a Quaker serving with Mennonite Central Committee. The tenor of his thesis is that science has become our god, and the *mechanistic* nature of medical research and treatment, rather than holistic health care, dominates in our technological culture. He draws theologically and philosophically on the contributions of Jacques Ellul, William Stringfellow and Ivan Illich. Downing, in regard to the first International Aids Conference held in Africa (2000), illustrates the political power of biomedicine by the contrasting explanations of the AIDS epidemic by South African president Thabo Mbeki (poverty, a socioeconomic factor) and the biomedical power structure (a virus)! Western media made a row of this, siding with the biomedical. Mbeki was ostracized.

God's role and the church's contribution to healing and health are often marginalized in modern health care. Desperately needed are creative alliances between health care practices and the church's healing ministry. We need a Christian view of health care, so that Christians whose vocation is professional health care see their health care work as part of their Christian calling.[15] This is what inspired the church (nineteenth-twentieth centuries) to send health care people all over the world as a witness to the gospel, in the tradition of Jesus' healing ministry proclaiming the advent of God's reign (see the end of chap. 8). Praying for the healing of the sick, with church elders and health care professionals in church, home or a health care facility, is part of holistic healing.

Also the lure of new health care technology must not "trump" other urgent needs in our communities. To illustrate: California's Proposition 71 was passed in 2004, authorizing sale of three billion dollars in bonds for stem cell research, while at the same time 3.8 million people were illiterate in the state.[16] Where we put our priorities is a social and moral issue. True, both of these are important, but important to whom? We must guard against catering to the desires of the wealthy while ignoring the needs of the poor.

2. *Scripture emphasizes justice, which occurs often in parallel to righteousness and shalom.* Justice was understood as compassion for the needy. Isaiah says,

> Is not this the fast that I choose:
>   to loose the bonds of *injustice*,
>   to undo the thongs of the yoke,
> to let the oppressed go free,
>   and to break every yoke?
> Is it not to share your bread with the hungry,

Citing also an earlier case (1848, in Illich) regarding use of antiseptic methods in childbirth by Dr. Ignaz Semmelweis that reduced postdelivery infection by fifteenfold, which was taken to implicate medical practice negatively, Downing asserts that "those in power are more concerned about the political power to name what is going on than the medical power to heal" (p. 69). See also Joel Shuman, "Naming Medicine Among the Powers," in Health and Healing, *Ex Auditu* 21 (2005): 52-66.

[15]Many doctors and nurses do. For a shining example of this see the article by Tim Leaman, "Hard Rock into Springs of Water: Working in Hope," *Mennonite Health Journal* 11, no. 3 (2009): 8-11, 22-26. Part of this appears in chap. 12.

[16]McDonough, *Can a Health Care Market Be Moral?* p. 179.

and bring the homeless poor into your house;
when you see the naked, to cover them,
    and not to hide yourself from your own kin?

Then your light shall break forth like the dawn,
    and your *healing* shall spring up quickly;
your vindicator shall go before you,
    the glory of the LORD shall be your rear guard.
Then you shall call, and the LORD will answer;
    you shall cry for help, and he will say, Here I am.

If you remove the yoke from among you,
    the pointing of the finger, the speaking of evil,
if you offer your food to the hungry
    and satisfy the needs of the afflicted,
then your light shall rise in the darkness
    and your gloom be like the noonday.
The LORD will guide you continually,
    and satisfy your needs in parched places,
    and make your bones strong;
and you shall be like a watered garden,
    like a spring of water, whose waters never fail.
        (Is 58:6-11, emphasis added)

Justice describes God's moral nature (Ps 89:14) and often occurs in parallel to righteousness (Ps 36:6; 72:1-2; Prov 2:9; 8:20; Is 5:7; 32:16; 33:5-6; 54:13-14; 60:17) or to shalom/peace (Is 32:16-17; 59:8; cf. Ps 85:10; Is 60:17). But the meaning of justice (*mishpat*) in Hebrew thought is not the same as the Greek view, popular in Western society, that each person receives *equal* due. In the biblical view justice means tending to the needs of the poor, widows, orphans and resident aliens (Ps 72:4, 12-14; 146:7-9; Is 10:1-2). We need to make health care accessible to all U.S. citizens, with compassion for the poor and resident aliens as well. This is a biblical moral imperative.[17]

Assisting the needy is linked often to *the fear of the Lord* (Deut 10:10-20; cf. Lev 19:14, 32; 25:17, 35-43; Is 33:5-6). Pursuit of justice in communal life is God's condition for living in the land God promised to the covenant

---

[17]See Ex 22:21-23; 23:6, 9; Lev 19:9-10, 34; Deut 10:18-19; 24:17-22; 26:12-13; cf. Prov 31:8-9; Is 1:17; 3:13-15; Amos 2:6-7; 8:4-6; and Jesus' healing the marginalized in chap. 3.

people: "Justice, and only justice, you shall pursue, so that you may live and occupy the land that the LORD your God is giving you" (Deut 16:20). Hear Amos also, "Let justice roll down like waters, / and righteousness like an ever flowing stream" (Amos 5:24).

The prophets raved and ranted because Israel failed to practice God's justice. Read the following texts and ponder their significance for health care access: Isaiah 5:5-10, Amos 8:4-10, Micah 6:1-8, and Nehemiah 5:1-13. These texts indicate that nothing stirs God's wrath against Israel more than failure to practice justice by caring for the needy. The same moral priority continues in the New Testament. James says, "Religion that is pure and undefiled before God, the Father, is this: to care for orphans and widows in their distress, and to keep oneself unstained by the world" (Jas 1:27).

The Isaiah 58 text is a well-known Lenten text, calling us to repent of our sinful ways. I suggest we link the health care issue to this Lenten theme, as we seek to reform the broken health care system.[18] People of good will have provided alternatives to the current U.S. system. Volunteer health care professionals provide care for the uninsured, with pay on a greatly reduced and graduated scale in relation to income, as clients are able.[19] This doesn't fix our national system, but it provides an alternative, an opportunity and moral mandate for the church. I commend churches working together ecumenically to provide this alternative health care, and hope for more such services to emerge. Those not working in health care can pray for those involved in these alternative programs, for their energy, wisdom, discernment and compassionate care for those whom they serve. We might also assist these programs, for example, by providing transportation for those who come to the health care centers.

The present health care system of the United States is a major departure from the church's history in health care (see chaps. 8 and 10). My neighbor nurse once emphatically said in our small group, "Putting profit ahead of actual health care is morally wrong. It is not Christian." In the early centuries and throughout the medieval period the church provided health care with no fees (see chap. 8)!

---

[18]See chap. 12 for such attempts modeled in several medical centers.

[19]The Center for Healing and Hope, in both Elkhart and Goshen, Indiana, is exemplary. Beginning in fall 2011 my congregation became a site for this service for the uninsured (see appendix 2). Similar services have emerged in other towns and cities—Iowa City, Iowa, for example.

Justice is a crucial matter in health care priorities. How is it that we spend millions on developing and advertising various meds for male sexual potency (Viagra, Cialis, etc.) while our research funding and efforts have not yet turned up a cure for malaria, an illness from which millions die every year in poorer countries of the world? How is it that the annual world defense budget is $1.2 trillion, while the global humanitarian assistance to the poor is $104 billion?[20] Just one week's global military spending could eradicate world hunger.[21] What are our moral priorities?

3. Jesus modeled health care inclusion of the poor and marginalized. Passion for health care is rooted in desire to be disciples of Jesus, who healed the sick as a sign of God's reign, challenged unjust societal structures and called for fundamental social change (Mk 11:15-19; Mt 9:35; Lk 7:18-23; 19:42). Judeo-Christian thought holds that every person has irreducible dignity and worth because they are created in God's image (Gen 1:26-27, 31). Judeo-Christian faith affirms life and health as God's gifts to which we respond in grateful stewardship (Ps 30:11-12). Love for God entails care for our neighbor's well-being (Mt 22:36-40; 25:34-40).

Christianity has done much to provide health care for people over the centuries (chap. 8). In the early centuries the church cared for the sick and the needy (chaps. 7-8). In recent centuries virtually all church denominations have sent many health care personnel overseas to serve human health needs (chap. 8). What is the church's moral responsibility to advocate and assist in health care changes, in light of the fifty million U.S. citizens who lack health care insurance, at least until 2014?

A key issue in the United States' broken health care system is *access.* Jesus' healing ministry had an unusual access policy. A third of those healed were socially ostracized: lepers, Gentiles and "sinners." Several were non-Israelites: the Syrophoenician woman and the centurion's son. For Jesus there were no exclusions, though lack of faith in Jesus as one sent

[20]Richard Stearns, *The Hole in Our Gospel* (Nashville: Thomas Nelson, 2009), p. 158.
[21]Stearns's figure was accessed July 2008, for 2007 spending. For 2010 it was $1.6 trillion. The World Food Summit estimates that $30 billion a year could eradicate world hunger. That is the amount of global military spending in a single week. See Anup Shah, "World Military Spending," *Global Issues,* May 2, 2011, www.globalissues.org/article/75/world-military-spending, and "Global Day of Action on Military Spending," Passionists International, April 5, 2011, http://passionistsinternational.wordpress.com/2011/04/05/global-day-of-action-on-military-spending.

from God with a special identity and mission hindered his ministry. When we consider the social, economic and political profile of the people Jesus healed, we learn an important lesson about health care access for today: the U.S. health care system needs much improvement, with more equal distribution patterns. Especially onerous is the "exclusion" policy for pre-existing conditions and canceling policies when clients are faced with major illness (hopefully now ended if the current health care bill continues to rule it illegal). This has been a form of triage, determined not by urgency of need but by the almighty dollar. The effect of this policy on our society takes its toll when unemployment is high. When a person is unemployed and loses health insurance, he or she is often only one health crisis away from home foreclosure or bankruptcy. Is it right to value the profit motive over a person's shalom?

Jesus taught his disciples to love all people, even enemies (Mt 5:43-48; Lk 6:27-36). Jesus' indiscriminate love command means abolishing exclusionary policies. It provides the biblical basis for seeking to make health care accessible for all.

Some churches are realizing anew that we can provide health care for all church employees only if we do it together as congregations, churchwide agencies and church-related institutions. But this is only a partial vision. We must extend the vision to provide health care for all, with the church supporting government initiatives that seek to accomplish that goal. The church is a body with interdependent members, so that the health and wellness of each member is the concern of all.[22]

4. *Sharing material resources is a basic teaching and practice of the New Testament church.* This point is the focus of chapter seven, but belongs in this five-point outline.

---

[22]The Mennonite Church USA Delegate Assembly in its 2007 meeting in San José took up this challenge: to provide a health care insurance/mutual aid program which would provide health care for all Mennonite pastors, of whom about a fourth had no health care insurance. In a delegate action the church resolved to do something about the problem of uninsured pastors. Conferences and congregations are recognizing that when the church does not provide health insurance for its workers it is compromising the church's witness to government and its witness before a watching world. This resolution provides the opportunity for the church to renew its practice of mutual aid. Scripture calls us to consider this as our responsibility to one another in the body of Christ. The plan is named "the Corinthian Plan" (see Amy Frykholm, "Healthcare Option: A Mennonite Plan for Mutual Aid," *Christian Century*, September 22, 2009, pp. 28-31). The plan was accepted tentatively at the July 2009 Delegate Assembly, and has now been adopted and implemented.

5. *Christian churches in the early centuries provided health care not only for their members but also for those outside the church, risking their own health.* The early Christians gave generously in resources, even their lives, to alleviate the horrific socioeconomic poverty and poor health conditions pervasive throughout the Roman Empire. This reality was the ugly underside of the boasted prosperity of the empire, the Pax Romana (see chap. 7). Chapter eight describes the early church's vast ministry to the poor and suffering.

LIVING TOWARD THE VISION

Attending to these five biblical themes and early Christian practices intensifies Christian concern for the U.S. health care system. We live in a society where high-tech health care innovations are abundant, often in overlapping availability and competing for the same demographic groups. Yet skewed distribution of resources, ever-rising expectations at both the beginning and end of life, and a for-profit, market-driven system, deprive the needy of health care. This is not shalom wellness for many people.

The late Dr. Willard Krabill described the situation exacerbating the health care crisis with the image of a "devil's triangle": in which quality, low cost and access compete against each other.

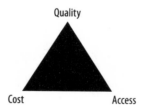

Figure 6.1. Devil's triangle

Krabill reported that many argue that only by sacrificing *quality* can *costs* be contained and *access* improved. Or only by sacrificing *access* is it possible to maintain *quality* and reasonable *costs*. Or if *costs* are lowered, then *quality* is compromised and the uninsured are not served. Krabill counters this view, however, maintaining that all three (high quality, access for all and low cost) are possible, if we

• accept restraint on high-tech procedures and medical fees

- lower lawyers' fees in malpractice suits (with fewer of them)

- convert insurance from economic gain to wider coverage benefits

- break the stranglehold of costly medications and medical equipment[23]

In the context of present health care practices another "move" might be added to this list:

- reduce the number of costly tests prescribed to gain cost-efficiency

Are any of these likely to happen? Perhaps they will, to a limited extent.[24]

While some gains have been made, the complexity of the U.S. health care industry makes the third change Krabill called for most unlikely. Insurance companies, with their fiduciary responsibility to shareholders to show good profits, are not likely to be financially gracious in medical payments for the insured. Every payment adds up on their loss ledger and thus impedes the growth goal of its profits.

As long as market-driven insurance companies control health care, hope for providing health care for the poor must come from other quarters (see efforts in chap. 12 and appendix 2). The Christian moral vision opposes policies that exclude those who need health care most. We need new lenses, not the "Devil's triangle," but "God's shalom triangle" (see fig. 6.2).

In contrast to the competitive nature of one against two in the Devil's triangle, God's shalom triangle models a cooperative relationship among all three components. Each enhances the others. God's shalom triangle

---

[23]Dr. Krabill presented this triangle-concept then afloat in health care literature in a plenary discussion at Mennonite Medical and Mennonite Nurses Associations' annual meetings in Atchison, Kan., June 24-27, 1993. For his answer to this notion, similar to the above, see Willard S. Krabill, M.D., "The church and national health care reform," *Mennonite Medical Messenger* 44, no. 3 (July–September, 1993): 7-18, especially pp. 8, 13-15. See also Krabill's article, "The Church Confronts Its Mission in Health and Healing" (unpublished manuscript, 1992). Available in Mennonite Historical Library, Goshen College, Goshen, Ind.

[24]We have seen some new initiatives, e.g., Walmart's and Target's initiative in 2006 to offer 300+ generic meds for $4 each per month or $10 per quarter. Other pharmacies soon followed suit, with making some antibiotics available free. This has been a big help to many people, but it does not solve the unaffordable prices of many other drugs for the uninsured. One way to solve this problem would be for the federal government to cap pharmaceutical costs, similar to the way Medicare and insurance companies negotiate with the pharmaceutical industry capping costs of prescription drugs. But then a further issue arises: will the rising *cost* of Medicaid and Medicare, and now Part D, change government policies?

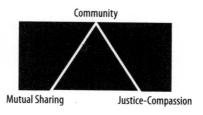

Figure 6.2. God's shalom triangle

introduces a counterpoint to each of the elements in the Devil's triangle, as follows:

Devil's	God's
Quality	Community
Costs	Mutual sharing
Access	Justice-compassion

Community is important for discernment and moral, spiritual support during times of hard decisions: for example, what procedures should be undertaken? Further, when people go through difficult health situations, the quality of medical care is supplemented by a caring community that brings encouragement, comfort and prayer to those experiencing the health crisis as well as to the family and close friends of that person. This can make a significant difference in the healing process. In this way *quality* is not measured only in medical terms but is enhanced by the community factor.

Similarly, the spiraling costs of health care call for community initiatives to meet costs through practice of *mutual aid*. This assumes that in God's shalom triangle stewardship of resources ranks high in value. Stewardship is a biblical value and moral priority that relates to all categories in the two triangles.[25] It enables the practice of *mutual aid*. Most insurance policies have high deductibles and thus leave those insured with high costs, some collateral necessities (living in facilities nearby, hospitals away from home, travel expenses) and many other related expenses. Living in God's shalom triangle means communities of care practice *mutual aid* to meet financial needs. See chapter seven for extended treatment of mutual aid.

[25]Both stewardship and community are prime values in Dr. Krabill's assessment of the church's mission in resolving the health care dilemma, ibid., 1993, p. 10. On stewardship see Willard M. Swartley, "Biblical Sources of Stewardship," in *The Earth Is the Lord's: Essays on Steward-ship*, ed. Mary Evelyn Jegen and Bruno V. Manno (New York: Paulist Press, 1978), pp. 22-43.

Further, justice-compassion combined with community will creatively initiate ways to provide access for all, a pressing issue in our time (see the "Justice" section in this chapter). As appendix two demonstrates, 20-25 percent of the people in a given local area may be without any insurance. How can communities of care respond to these needs? The Center for Healing and Hope is one such model that may be duplicated in communities across the nation.

One factor that makes health care expensive is the *fear* factor underlying the system. Physicians fear malpractice suits and thus tend to order more tests than deemed necessary, thus practicing "defensive" medicine to protect themselves. Malpractice insurance costs continue to spiral; this in turn increases physicians' fees. Patients *fear* they won't get what they want and become demanding and are often ungrateful for the good services they receive. Their demands increase health care costs and then insurance companies raise their premiums to protect themselves from increasing losses, in light of these combined fear factors. One important contribution from God's shalom triangle is to puncture this cycle of fear. Reminding us that God's presence dispels fear, the teaching of the churches, synagogues and mosques can help replace fear with gratitude. This will affect the climate of the health care system, a most important contribution of God's shalom triangle by those who cultivate these virtues in their lives.

If we embrace these biblical values, we can break the grip of the devil's triangle and find the peace and joy of living in God's shalom triangle. To do this we need to be committed and creative, using our wealth and church personnel resources to find ways to include the excluded. If insurance systems in our society are not able to deliver, church-based initiatives are necessary to shift triangle dominion: from the devil's "lenses" to God's.

> God Almighty, you revealed yourself as
>   YHWH-*rapha:* LORD who heals,
>   YHWH-*shalom:* LORD who gives peace.
> Look upon us in judgment and mercy,
>   for we cry to you for healing and peace.
> Let us know health and wholeness
>   despite our sorrows and sicknesses.
> Heal us, and we shall be healed,
>   save us and we shall be saved.

Wounded for our sins and transgressions,
    restore to us your healing shalom
    and the joy of your salvation.

In the name of the great Physician, Jesus Christ,
Amen.

Willard Swartley

7

❖

Biblical and Theological (Anabaptist) Foundations of Health Care Through Mutual Aid

God created our [human] race for sharing [koinonia] . . .
making it common [koinos] to all humans,
and creating all things for all. . . .
Therefore all things are common . . .
and let not the rich claim more than the rest.

Clement of Alexandria

Mutual aid is one of the foundational practices of the Christian faith. John Gager and William Walsh and John Langan say,

> Early Christianity['s] survival, growth, and success [depended on] "a single, overriding internal factor," namely, a "radical sense of Christian community—open to all, insistent on absolute loyalty, and concerned for every aspect of the believer's life. From the very beginning, the one distinctive gift of Christianity was this sense of community."[1]

> Further, "an essential part of this sense of community depended on the willingness of Christians to aid those in need and on the teachings of the Christian church with regard to the right use of material goods."[2]

---

[1]John Gager, *Kingdom and Community: The Social World of Early Christianity* (Englewood Cliffs, N.J.: Prentice-Hall, 1976), p. 140.

[2]William Walsh and John Langan, "Patristic Social Consciousness: The Church and the Poor," in *The Faith That Does Justice: Examining the Christian Sources for Social Change*, ed. John C. Haughey (New York: Paulist Press, 1977), p. 113.

Community and mutual aid were twin pillars undergirding the early Christians' survival and growth. Strongly bonded communities form the matrix for mutual aid, enabling cost-sharing for health care (witness the Amish and Hutterite communities, and to a lesser extent contemporary Mennonite and Seventh-day Adventist churches as well; see appendix 1). Based on the accounts of sharing of resources in Acts 2:43-47 and Acts 4:32-37, and later the relief gift for the saints in Jerusalem (Acts 11:27-29; Rom 15:25-28), we may conclude that when the Holy Spirit guides community life, the community will practice mutual aid. John Howard Yoder relates care for the poor to participation in the Eucharist. He emphasizes that breaking bread in Acts 2:46 is to be joined to "There was not a needy person among them" (Acts 4:34). Breaking bread means "sharing with one another . . . ordinary day-to-day material sustenance." Thus, "the Eucharist is an economic act. To do rightly the practice of breaking bread together is a matter of economic ethics."[3]

I offer a pictorial guide, figure 7.1, to grasp the biblical and theological thinking that makes mutual aid a fundamental practice of Christian living.

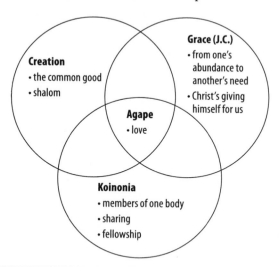

Figure 7.1. Biblical and theological foundations of and motivations for mutual aid in early Christianity

[3]John Howard Yoder develops this point in discussing the Lord's Supper under the title "Disciples Break Bread Together" (*Body Politics: Five Practices of the Christian Community Before the Watching World* [Scottdale, Penn.: Herald Press, 1992], p. 21; see pp. 14-27).

This figure puts *agapē* love at the center, reflecting what was central in early Christian experience, "Behold how they love one another." Mutual aid is a practical expression of that love. Indeed, Origen in the second century defended Christianity against Celsus's charge—that Christians are wicked—by pointing to their "generosity and sharing [*koinōnikon*]." Even the unbelievers saw this as proof against wickedness.[4]

The three circles that interconnect flow out of *agapē* love, empowering practical expression of mutual aid and health care practice. Mutual aid is on a human level grounded in creation theology, as humans are created in God's image: "God has implanted the principle of mutual aid into the very nature of creation."[5] We therefore seek to become stewards of our resources with the same generosity evident in the beauty and wealth of God's creation. This contrasts to consumption and conservation. Consumption is wasteful. Conservation makes us frugal and often self-protective in the face of need. Either may feed on selfishness. But true creation theology means we generously help others because God has been generous to us in the bounties and beauty of his creation. Living selfishly deprives the community of shalom. Mutual aid, given out of a generous, loving heart enables shalom to flourish. In applying this point to mutual aid we need to ask how policies help people, and also how policies hurt people. Consuming abundant resources *we* have while *others* are in need usually hurts more than helps.

Anabaptist practice of mutual aid makes the point. In 1528 in the city of Augsburg, Germany, prospective Anabaptist members were asked, "If need should require it, are you prepared to devote all your possessions to the service of the brotherhood, and do you agree not to fail any member that is in need if you are able to help?"[6] This is a radical promise as part of church membership: to practice mutual aid, in giving and receiving.

[4]Justo L. González, *Faith and Wealth: A History of Early Christian Ideas on the Origin, Significance, and Use of Money* (San Francisco: Harper & Row, 1990), pp. 118-19; *Contra Celsus* 3.78.
[5]J. Winfield Fretz, cited in Cornelius A. Buller, "Mutual Aid: Harbinger of the Kingdom?" in *Building Communities of Compassion*, ed. Willard M. Swartley and Donald B. Kraybill (Scottdale, Penn: Herald Press, 1998), p. 81. Buller begins by appeal to human creation in God's image. The flowering of mutual aid practice, however, flows out of God's kingdom vision with trinitarian love relationships as its theological foundation. *Agapē* love motivates Christian practice, which in turn is a harbinger of God's perfected kingdom (ibid., pp. 83-92).
[6]Jeni Heitt Umble, "Mutual Aid Among the Augsburg Anabaptists," in *Building Communities of Compassion*, ed. Willard M. Swartley and Donald B. Kraybill (Scottdale, Penn.: Herald Press., 1998), p. 115.

Baptism initiates one into mutual aid. Teaching the practice of mutual aid belongs in the catechism of those preparing for baptism.

The second circle points to *grace* as foundation and motivation for mutual aid. In Greek the word for "grace gift" is *charis*, from which we get the word *charismatic*. Paul uses *charis* as the basis for mutual aid. It's the big point in 2 Corinthians 8-9. "Grace" (*charis*) is used ten times in these two chapters. The first use speaks of God's action and initiative for us in Jesus Christ: "We want you to know, brothers and sisters, about the grace of God" (2 Cor 8:1). At the end of the appeal Paul returns to grace/thanksgiving to God: "Thanks (*charis*) be to God for his indescribable gift" (2 Cor 9:15). The eight uses between these bookends focus on the horizontal movement of the grace.

In these eight uses of *charis* we have a persuasive basis for mutual aid, with seven strands of rationale:

1. It is an expression of God's grace (8:1-24).

2. It proves the genuineness of one's love (8:8, 24).

3. It expresses the fruit of the Spirit (8:7-8).

4. It follows the example of Jesus Christ, who, "though he was rich . . . became poor" (8:9).

5. It works toward equality (8:13-15).

6. It is to be done generously (8:2) and cheerfully (9:7), with assurance that the Lord will multiply the giver's resources (9:8-10).

7. It is a ministry that meets the needs of other saints (9:12-13).

In Romans 12:8 three gifts of grace are expressed in similar forms of sharing: "he who contributes, in liberality; he who gives aid, with zeal; he who does acts of mercy, with cheerfulness" (rsv).[7]

In his gospel mission *apostle* Paul also does the work of the *deacon*, collecting aid for the poor in Jerusalem, the need that occasions Paul's passionate plea. Paul speaks of this relief gift in Romans 15 at length and grounds it in "the grace given me by God" (Rom 15:15). He prays that this

---

[7]The translation is markedly different in the nrsv: "the giver, in generosity; the leader, in diligence; the compassionate, in cheerfulness." While *proistamenous* can indeed mean "leader" (one who leads), as well as giving aid in deacon-type ministry, the cluster of financially related terms supports the rsv interpretation.

"offering of the Gentiles may be acceptable, sanctified by the Holy Spirit" (Rom 15:16). Later Paul describes the effort more fully:

> At present, however, I am going to Jerusalem in a ministry to the saints; for Macedonia and Achaia have been pleased to share their resources with the poor among the saints at Jerusalem. They were pleased to do this, and indeed they owe it to them; for if the Gentiles have come to share in their spiritual blessings, they ought also to be of service to them in material things. (Rom 15:25-27)

This mutuality, or "mutualism," as Justin Meggitt describes it,[8] arises from the peace bond within the communities of faith, especially between the Gentile and Jewish Christians, central to Paul's view of justification and reconciliation as the essential core of God's saving work in Jesus Christ. Mutual care for one another is not only an important manifestation of the gift of grace within Paul himself and in the community, but it is also evidence that the formerly alienated people are now one in Jesus Christ who is their peace (Eph 2:14). Practicing mutual aid to enable health care for all is *peacemaking*, a crucial element in one's experience of shalom. Meggitt identifies two characteristics of this mutual sharing:

> Firstly, it was aimed at promoting *material well being*. It was initially undertaken to achieve a tangible end: *the relief of the economically poor in the Jerusalem church.* . . . Secondly, it was thoroughly *mutual* in its character. *It was in no sense an individual or unilateral undertaking for any of those involved.* Paul emphasizes that *all* the members were contributors as, indeed, were *all* the communities (we hear of no exceptions). It was not intended to be the work of a few wealthy members or congregations.[9]

Meggitt further notes that such assistance, because it was *mutual*, would be expected to be returned when and if the situation of need were reversed.

---

[8]Justin J. Meggitt, *Paul, Poverty and Survival* (Edinburgh: T & T Clark, 1998), pp. 157-64. For monograph studies of Paul's collection for the poor in Jerusalem see Keith F. Nickle, *The Collection: A Study in Paul's Strategy*, Studies in Biblical Theology 48 (London: SCM Press, 1966); Dieter Georgi, *Remembering the Poor: The History of Paul's Collection for Jerusalem*, trans. John Bowden (Nashville: Abingdon, 1992).

[9]Meggitt, *Paul, Poverty and Survival*, p. 159. Meggitt's thesis as a whole, appealing to primary sources on the economic realities of the first century, is that Paul and the churches he founded belonged to the 99 percent of the population's poor people; they shared generously from their limited means. This fits with Paul's profuse appeal to *grace* in 2 Cor 8–9.

This expresses true care for another, sustaining shalom in its fullest sense in communities of faith.

Paul regarded this mutual aid as proof of the unity between Jews and Gentile believers in Jesus Christ. Hence he willingly gave his life for the cause, despite prophetic declaration that he would encounter arrest and imprisonment in Jerusalem (Acts 21:7-14). Paul says, "I am ready not only to be bound but even to die in Jerusalem for the name of the Lord Jesus" (v. 13). Paul regarded this relief gift to Jerusalem as the crowning achievement of his apostolic call, certifying that Gentile and Jewish messianic believers are truly one in Jesus Christ, peace fellows through the blood of the cross of the Lord Jesus Christ. The peace of the cross expresses itself concretely in mutual care for one another. Mutual aid is not an add-on to the gospel. Like peacemaking, it is an essential core of the gospel, a chief characteristic of koinonia.

In the seventeenth century wealthy Dutch Anabaptists sent mutual aid money to the impoverished and persecuted Swiss Anabaptists. In the 1630s, 1660s and again in the 1690s the Dutch gave huge amounts of aid, over a half-million guilders. In the early years of Swiss Anabaptism, giving aid to fellow Anabaptists became a point in the trials leading to torture and sometimes death. Giving shelter, food, drink or secret refuge was cause for arrest. Yes, mutual aid was a crime. Anabaptists knowingly risked their lives to do it. A shining testimony of love and commitment!

The third circle of love's commitment shows that mutual aid flows out of *koinonia*, a word difficult to translate adequately. Common translations of *koinonia* are fellowship, sharing, participation, members one of another. It means being glued together in Christ. The word describes basic aspects of Christian experience. Represented visually, George Panikulam utilizes a full-page cross with "Jesus Christ" diagonally across the cross's crossbars, "Father" over the whole, and "Call to *Koinōnia*" at the bottom (see fig. 7.2).[10] The top of the vertical bar represents koinonia in 1 John, indicating that koinonia is a key emphasis in 1 John, recurring often (see McDermond's commentary treatment of this theme).[11] The crossbar of the cross

---

[10]From George Panikulam, *Koinōnia in the New Testament: A Dynamic Expression of Christian Life*, Analecta Biblica 85 (Rome: Biblical Institute Press, 1979), p. 7.

[11]J. E. McDermond, *1, 2, 3 John*, Believers Church Bible Commentary (Scottdale, Penn: Herald Press, 2011), pp. 36, 45-46, 50-51, 54-55. The latter two sets of pages are brief topical discussions: one on "the text in biblical context" and the other, "the text in the life of the Church."

identifies koinonia in Acts, where it occurs crucially in the book's summaries (Acts 2:42-47; 4:32-35; 5:12-16). The long bottom part of the vertical crossbar has on both its sides numerous term connections that koinonia has in Paul's writings: sufferings, Eucharist, spirit, collection, gospel and faith. Various translations choose different English meanings in these associations (any of the four listed).

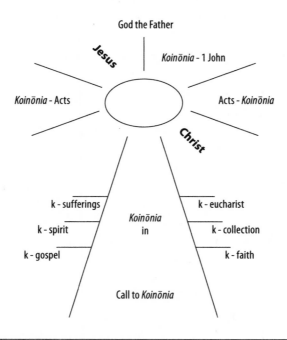

Figure 7.2. Centrality of koinonia in early Christianity

Koinonia extends into many dimensions of Christian belief and practice, as figure 7.2 shows. Mutual aid is a *practice* of Christian faith.[12] We cannot be corporately one in Christ without sharing materially to assist another's shalom. Koinonia marks the early Christian community's praising God daily in the temple and breaking bread in homes with joyful and generous

---

[12]The word *practice* as used in this chapter and appendix 1 has a fund of meaning behind it. It describes formation of virtues expressed in a spontaneous, consistent manner. For background explanation see Joseph J. Kotva Jr., "Mutual Aid as 'Practice,'" in *Building Communities of Compassion*, ed. Willard M. Swartley and Donald B. Kraybill (Scottdale, Penn.: Herald Press, 1998), pp. 57-79.

hearts. The wonders and signs done by the apostles lead to awe. Community need motivated this mutual practice in Acts. "Koinonia means first of all, not fellowship in the sense of good feelings toward each other, but sharing."[13]

Virtually everyone in the Roman Empire was poor (99 percent); only a few were wealthy. Likewise, the church was largely composed of poor people (1 Cor 1:26-28). By A.D. 251, the church in Rome had a massive program of care for widows and the poor. With numerous house churches throughout the city, fifteen hundred people were on the church's support role. Bishop Cornelius was aided by seven deacons, seven more subdeacons, and ninety-four more laypeople working in minor roles to aid the needy.[14] By mid-third century the growing Christian church had taken over the social welfare of its vast membership in an organized way. Deacons were essential in early Christianity, begun already in Acts 6:1-6 and even into twentieth-century practice of mutual aid. Churches might consider reestablishing the office of ordained or commissioned deacon in the congregation and restore this apostolic teaching.[15]

The early church's practice of mutual aid brilliantly enacted Paul's vision for the gospel: "that through the church the manifold wisdom of God might now be made known to the principalities and powers" (Eph 3:10 RSV). While the early church stressed aiding fellow members of the community, they also aided the poor outside the church. The peace of Jesus Christ expressed itself in the community's care for the poor and despised of the *plebs urbana*. Not only did the Christian community practice mutual aid among its own members, but it sought also to alleviate the horrific socioeconomic poverty conditions of the empire.[16] Early Christianity witnessed to Jesus Christ's victory over the powers by means of the church's incredible practice of charity and mutual aid.

---

[13]Justo González, *Faith and Wealth*, p. 83.

[14]Eusebius, *Ecclesiastical History* 6.43.11.

[15]As voiced by Mark Vincent, many lament that mutual aid has been compromised among Mennonites by two developments: the loss of deacons, with their work splintered into many other activities. Second, organizations that were started to strengthen and support mutual aid in the congregation are no longer vested in their priorities to promote mutual aid in congregational practice. Other interests or economic pressures have subverted them. This means that *koinonia*, *charis* and *shalom* have all been weakened. The restoration of the deacon, as an office, who oversees mutual aid and charity in the congregation ought to be a priority.

[16]For description of these dire conditions, see Meggitt, *Paul, Poverty and Survival*, pp. 41-73.

The Roman world treated human life with contempt in many instances, especially allowing female infants to die, with their bodies decaying in open sewers running down the middle of city streets. Rodney Stark, from his sociological study of early Christianity says, "We've unearthed sewers clogged with the bones of newborn girls." The early Christians "had to live with a trench running down the middle of the road, in which you could find dead bodies decomposing."[17] Christians did not put sewer systems in the cities, but they did speak against infanticide; they cared for each other and for the weak in a society that otherwise blinded itself to human need. Though agnostic in his personal stance toward Christianity, Stark is convinced that the early Christians made a striking difference in their world, by standing for life over against death, caring for each other and valuing women and children, granting them dignity and worth that manifested God's kingdom values amid an immoral degenerate social order.[18]

What can we do to restore what we have lost? How can we do better in sharing resources? One example is the late Bob Baker's "Fifties Club," which he began at Belmont Mennonite Church. Because a church member once gave him a $50 bill when his daughter and son-in-law with many children were financially pressed, he began this club to extend the favor toward others in need in the congregation.

Caring for the poor and conferring human dignity upon women and children became a powerful testimony to Jesus Christ that unmasked the illusions of the powers. When Constantine became emperor under the banner of his Christian conversion—though he was baptized only at his death—he took over the Christian charity patterns already developed,

---

[17]"A Double Take on Early Christianity: An Interview with Rodney Stark," interview by Mike Aquilina, in *Touchstone* 13, no. 1 (2000): 44, 47. For fuller treatment see Rodney Stark, *The Rise of Christianity: A Sociologist Reconsiders History* (Princeton, N.J.: Princeton University Press, 1996), esp. "Epidemics," pp. 76-94, and "Urban Chaos and Crisis," pp. 147-62. He says, outside "on the streets [was] mud, open sewers, manure, and crowds. In fact, human corpses—adult as well as infant—were sometimes just pushed into the street and abandoned" (ibid., p. 154). Stark also describes the Christian communities as caring for each other through networks of support and doing much to alleviate the plight of sufferers during plagues and amid horrid urban conditions. Yet their survival rates were higher than those of the general population.

[18]Stark, "A Double Take on Early Christianity," p. 47. For a contemporary act of loving care for a destitute person, repulsive in dirty body and odor, read E.R. nurse Dawn Husnick's care for such a person, cited by Scot McKnight in *A Community Called Atonement* (Nashville: Abingdon, 2007), pp. 3-4.

trying to maintain a welfare system. Certainly the life of the Christian community that enacts the new creation of the gospel of Jesus Christ will bear a positive peacemaking demonstration of how Christian faith and life orders society through love that shares resources to those in need, honoring the dignity of each human being. [19]

The Pauline metaphor of the church as a body, with its many dimensions of application—for example, "one body" of diverse origins (Eph 2:16; 4:4) and "one body" with many members (1 Cor 12:12-27)—is a strong ecclesiological image. If one member suffers, the whole body suffers. Theologically, the corporate image "body of Christ" is a firm foundation for sharing resources in times of need. Every aspect of koinonia in figure 7.2 gains depth of meaning when koinonia is viewed as the natural expression of being "one body." Mutual aid, then, is not a gospel add-on but a fundamental fruit of the "one body." To be truly Christ's body—indeed in the Eucharistic cup we drink (1 Cor 10:16-17)—means we will share our resources to aid the health and healing of the body, both physically and metaphorically as the people of God. Mutual aid demonstrates that we are *one body* of Christ and in Christ.

---

[19]For more on mutual aid, see Willard M. Swartley, "Mutual Aid Based in Jesus and Early Christianity," in *Building Communities of Compassion*, ed. Willard M. Swartley and Donald B. Kraybill (Scottdale, Penn.: Herald Press, 1998), pp. 21-39.

8

❖

Health Care in
Christian History and Mission

Early Christianity may be seen as a Jewish sect that had, as one of its
primary goals, the reformation of the health problems found in the health
care systems of Greco–Roman traditions. Far from being a marginal in-
terest, health care was part of the core of its mission and strategy for
gaining converts to this Jewish sect.

A variety of features afforded Christianity an advantage over its
many competitors. . . . The combination of benefits offered by the
Christian approach to health care was one of the primary factors in the
rise of Christianity.

Hector Avalos, *Health Care and the Rise of Christianity*

Christianity has a rich history of health care. From the first century to the
present, Christian response to the sick and dying lies at the heart of
Christian moral praxis (recall Jesus' healing ministry in chap. 3). The early
church's *practice* of caring for the sick and sharing with the poor and needy
looms large in the church's understanding of its calling and ministry.[1] The
church's growth depended largely on its health care component: mutual
aid or charity in caring for the sick (chap. 7).

---

[1] S. C. Muir connects this ministry with "love for one another," a prominent Johannine motif.
See his article "'Look How They Love One Another': Early Christian and Pagan Care of the
Sick and Other Charity," in *Religious Rivalries in the Early Roman Empire and the Rise of Chris-*
tianity, ed. L. E. Vaage (Waterloo, Ont.: Wilfrid Laurier University Press, 2006), pp. 213-32.
Note also Allen Verhey's chapter on this topic in *Remembering Jesus: Christian Community,*
Scripture, and the Moral Life (Grand Rapids: Eerdmans, 2002), pp. 117-32.

The good Samaritan parable (Lk 10:25-37) and Jesus' healing ministry inspired the early church. During the second and third centuries the early church continued to value health care as an aspect of its mission. Health care was integral to the church's mission. Amanda Porterfield documents this recurring emphasis in early Christianity:

> As a number of primary documents attest, care for the sick was a distinctive and remarkable characteristic of early Christian missionary outreach. Early Christians nursed the sick to emulate the healing ministry of Jesus, to express their faith in the ongoing healing power of Christ, and to distinguish Christian heroism in face of sickness and death from pagan fear. Polycarp, bishop of Smyrna, in the early second century, identified care of the sick as one of the chief tasks for which church elders were responsible. A guidebook for Christian communities written in Rome around 215 instructed bishops to pay house calls on sick members.[2]

Porterfield cites historian R. J. S. Barrett-Lennard's study of fourth-century Egyptian papyri. Written by lay Christians, these early letters mention illness and concern for the sick much more often than the letters written by pagans. A key difference between the two cohorts of letters is that "the surviving letters written by Christians explicitly refer to God and Christ as gods concerned about human illness and healing."[3] To document further this distinctive feature of early Christianity, Porterfield cites similar conclusions from Stanley Harakas's study of holy men in the early centuries. Dionysius, third-century bishop of Alexandria, Egypt, describes the dedication and fearlessness of Christians in caring for the sick, especially those infected with contagious diseases. Dionysius writes, "people without Christian faith 'pushed away those with the first signs of the disease and fled from their dearest. They even threw them half dead into the roads and treated unburied corpses like refuse in hopes of avoiding the plague of death.'"[4] Indeed, the early Christians ministered heroically.

Hector Avalos, often critical of Christianity and its claims, describes the health care system of early Christianity extensively (see the epigraph of this chap.). Avalos integrates the young science of medical anthropology

---

[2]Amanda Porterfield, *Healing in the History of Christianity* (Oxford: Oxford University Press, 2005), p. 47.
[3]Ibid., p. 48.
[4]Ibid., p. 49.

with biblical studies, noting especially John Pilch's anthropological contributions to healing in the New Testament.[5] Avalos's method emphasizes
"health care *systems*," considering such interrelated factors as the patient's
religious or social status, whether the prescribed therapeutic structure is
simple or complex, sufficiency of faith and prayer for healing, the cost of
health care, the access factor, and the degree of temporal restrictions.[6]

In a comparative grid of Christianity's health care system to other contemporary religious systems (Asclepius, Isis, secular Greco-Roman, Le-
vitical), Christianity had a definite edge. Social or religious status did not
affect the outcome or complicate the process. The therapeutic prescription
was simple, not complex. Faith and prayer were efficacious. The Christians' health care was free—in contrast to all the other systems. Location,
mobility and waiting time were not prohibitive. There were no access
problems. Avalos amply demonstrates the health care benefits of early
Christianity.

In concluding his study Avalos, like Stark (chap. 7), claims that Christianity's health care system was its major reason for rapid growth within
the Roman Empire, where other health care systems were too complex,
expensive or restrictive in other ways. In the third century Origen proclaimed Christ as the "physician of souls." In the next century Basil, who
studied Hippocratic texts, said God gave medicine, for which people
should be grateful, though he declared also that the soul outweighs the
body in our temporal care and concern—hence asceticism toward bodily
desires and needs.[7]

The early church remembered Jesus as healer proclaiming the kingdom

---

[5]Hector Avalos, *Health Care and the Rise of Christianity* (Peabody, Mass.: Hendrickson,
1999), pp. 24-26. Pilch in turn utilizes Mary Douglas's anthropological purity-unclean categories. See also Avalos's study of pre-Christian cultures in the ancient Near Eastern cultures,
in *Illness and Health Care in the Ancient Near East: The Role of the Temple in Greece, Mesopotamia,
and Israel*, Harvard Semitic Monographs 54 (Atlanta: Scholars Press, 1995). In ancient cultures, health care was associated with religion (often temples). Avalos begins his 1999 book
with the story of Mexican Catholic Maria Atkinson (1879-1963) seeking healing for her cancer. After months of seeking answers in the American Southwest through alternative healing
efforts, she finally found her answer and cure in Pentecostal prayer and anointing with oil.
Avalos cites this story to introduce the topic of his book, showing that early Christianity's healing powers continued into the twentieth century. Atkinson began the Mexican branch of the
Church of God (headquartered in Cleveland, Tenn.), which as of 1999 numbered 53,000.
[6]Avalos, *Health Care*, pp. 117-19.
[7]Ibid., p. 53.

of God drawing near. The church continued these dual aspects of Jesus' ministry. Several recent studies have focused on the portrait of early Christian missionaries cast also in the role of physicians. Bazzana concludes that the early Christian pattern was to some extent a mimesis of Greco-Roman medical doctors but also cultural criticism of the same, for in the empire-society doctors in the West received both a societal "tax" (*iatrikon*) and fee for service (*misthos*). In the East a (generous) salary was often forfeited in exchange for prestige and honor in the community. While the Christian healing/kingdom proclamation resembles in some ways the physician model, it also critiqued that system by refusing fees for healing. Hospitality for the itinerant missionaries (food and lodging) though, was expected as well as honor from those who were recipients of the itinerant's healings.[8]

With Christianity's paradigm shift in the Constantinian era, health care continued as a priority of the church, but it became more institutionalized and complex.

HEALTH CARE IN THE MEDIEVAL PERIOD

Epidemics continued to ravage ancient cities, and new levels of organized health care developed in response. Constantinople, center of Eastern Christianity, paved the way in the development of hospitals. As Roth writes regarding the Christian legacy,

> Already in 325, the Council of Nicaea commanded that a building dedicated to the care of the sick be constructed in every cathedral town. The hospice of St. Basil at Caesarea in Cappadocia, for example, completed by 370, was renowned for its treatment of the sick and as a place of refuge for travelers and poor people.
>
> Early Christians built similar hospices at Constantinople and Alexandria in Egypt and in cities throughout Syria and Asia Minor.[9]

---

[8]Giovanni Battista Bazzana, "Early Christian Missionaries as Physicians: Healing and its Cultural Value in the Greco-Roman Context," *Novum Testamentum* 51 (2009): 232-51. Drawing on Pilch's and Horsley's studies of such healers in the sociocultural context of the time, these "physicians" would be classified in the "folk" category rather than the "popular" or "professional" (ibid., p. 247).
[9]John D. Roth, "The Christian and Anabaptist Legacy in Healthcare," in *Healing Healthcare: A Study and Action Guide on Healthcare Access in the United States*, ed. Joseph J. Kotva Jr. (Scottdale, Penn.: Faith & Life Resources, 2005), p. 13.

Christian physicians were proactive in developing cordial and natural ties between medicine and Christian faith. In 411-412 Syrian bishop Rabbula of Edessa sought to bring common vision to the many churches in Edessa—often battling each other over doctrine—through the Christian mission of constructing hospitals to care for the sick. By the sixth century an important school was established at Nisibis, along the Silk Road, with a department of medicine. "Nestorian priests and merchants also took their [medical] learning to China, converting members of the Uighur tribe in the eighth century. One famous general in the Chinese army during the eighth century was a Nestorian priest known for healing and caring for the poor."[10]

In the next centuries, "an age replete with violence, bloodshed, blindness, crippled limbs, and festering sores, Christianity advanced in Europe . . . as a popular aid to human recovery, strength, and vitality."[11] One venue carrying forward early Christian healing practice was the emergence of special saints as agents of, and sacred relics possessing, miraculous healing power. Beliefs in the healing power of the bones of certain saints led to grave diggings to treasure the bones of those saints, for example, Oswald, the Christian king of North Umbria, England.[12] Numerous healing miracles lace this period of the church's history, blending pagan and Christian practices, integrated with current medical practice.

Hildegard of Bingen, a twelfth-century German Benedictine, developed a "proto-science" of medicine. Familiar with Latin texts based on Greek medical thought, she "compiled two medical works: *Causes and Cures*, a depiction of and explanation of the origins and remedies of numerous diseases, and *Physica*, a nine-book pharmacopoeia." These works contain "extensive knowledge of herbs and their medicinal uses and pioneering attention to gynecological processes and problems."[13] A Renaissance humanist several centuries later commends Hildegard for "her knowledge of 'the many wonders and secrets of nature.'"[14]

In the medieval centuries healing and monastic life readily blended. In some monastic communities hospitals, including pharmacies, were part of

---

[10]Porterfield, *Healing in the History of Christianity*, p. 52.
[11]Ibid., p. 69.
[12]Ibid., pp. 69-70. Porterfield here draws on Bede's eighth-century history of the church.
[13]Porterfield, *Healing in the History of Christianity*, pp. 73-74.
[14]Ibid., p. 75.

the structural layout, along with chapel, kitchen and other facilities. "In Eastern Christianity, healing shrines and hospitals were often built alongside each other, and the cooperation between the two was fairly routine." Patients might go to the hospital first and be referred to the saints, or the reverse order might also occur. While cooperation was common, rivalry between the two also existed. Ambivalent toward Greek scientific medicine, several popes issued edicts proscribing certain medical practices. "By the early twelfth century, Catholic monks had become so proficient and specialized in medical arts that church councils banned them from practicing medicine for gain and pursuing medical studies outside of religious centers and outside the context of religious charity."[15] Not until the modern period is medicine perceived as a secular pursuit, apart from the church's jurisdiction. Attaching healing to penance and indulgences unfortunately set the stage for the Reformers' reaction to much the medieval church exemplified regarding health care as the church's prerogative within the state-church context.

THE MODERN PERIOD

Both Calvin and Luther reacted strongly to the Roman Catholic practices of attaching healing power to saints, relics and petitioners' healing prayers addressed to Mary. Because penance, indulgences and even baptism had all been associated with healing in Catholicism, the Reformers were mostly negative to healing. Within an ever-growing emphasis on individualism, the Reformers linked salvation to the spiritual experience of the believer, privileging soul and spirit over the body. At the same time the Reformers sought to restore the early church's purity, with divine providence (Calvin), salvation by faith alone (Luther), and the dawning of God's kingdom as of prime importance. Human suffering, said Calvin, is to be viewed more pedagogically, "as a means of teaching, testing, and drawing men and women toward him [God]."[16] Luther, however, held a more positive view toward human health and medicine, basing his view on God's creation. He emphasized more than Calvin the need for believers to

---

[15]Ibid., pp. 79-80.

[16]Ibid., p. 101. While this might seem to be a harsh judgment on Calvin, a biography of Calvin, Alister E. McGrath's *A Life of John Calvin*, does not contravene the judgment. On the one hand, his contribution is primarily a "religion of the book" devoted to orthodoxy (p. 181). His social influence mentions nothing of concern for suffering and physical welfare (pp. 188-93).

care for the body, for it too was created by God.[17]

The Reformers' devaluing of health care in reaction to Catholicism led to major shifts in church priorities,[18] so much so that a hospital crisis developed in certain areas of Western Christianity. This decline of religious support for health care was "especially calamitous in England, where Henry VIII confiscated church properties, including hospitals and many pilgrimage shrines, in an effort to sever England's ties to Rome. . . . Henry dissolved five hospitals." Two hospitals continued to operate and two more were founded by 1560, "one during Edward VI's reign and another by the authority of Catholic Queen Mary."[19]

Drawing on the Reformers' and Renaissance's new thought and freedom, the early modern era emphasized individual and private freedom, with budding insights into psychology. Science developed in this period, in embryonic stage, laying the foundation for what later would become a rift between science and religion, with science assaulting religious beliefs. Development of secular thought freed science from religion and also led to a bankruptcy of the earlier synthesis of Christianity and healing. Porterfield's assessment of this development merits pondering:

> Some might claim that both medical science and social welfare advanced because Christianity retreated to a more private sphere [with the advent of Protestantism]; others would argue that the healing traditions associated with ancient and medieval Christianity do not come off badly in comparison with the inhumanities of managed care and endemic poverty in the world today. However the pluses and minuses of modernization are calculated, Christianity's long-standing investment in healing and attention to suffering persisted in the context of new discoveries in scientific medicine and new approaches to health care, and also contributed to those new dis-

---

[17]Porterfield, *Healing in the History of Christianity*, p. 111.

[18]Anabaptists also reacted against certain Catholic practices, though they continued health care in their communities. "In many communities, Anabaptists gained local renown for their skills as midwives, physicians, or healers. In Moravia, for example, Hutterite physicians often found employment in the courts of local lords. . . . Anabaptist-Mennonites as a persecuted minority, gravitate[d] to the healing arts" (Roth, "The Christian and Anabaptist Legacy in Healthcare," p. 14). Miracles of healing—even resurrections—occurred among Anabaptists as well (see Stuart Murray, *Biblical Interpretation in Anabaptist Perspective* [Scottdale, Penn.: Herald Press, 2000], pp. 133-34). Reacting to the Catholic "anointing with oil" as an ordinance of last rites, Mennonites did not practice anointing with oil for healing until the nineteenth and twentieth centuries (see p. 80 n. 39).

[19]Porterfield, *Healing in the History of Christianity*, pp. 109-10.

coveries and approaches. Long-standing connections between Christianity, healing, and health care passed into the modern era, even as the practice of each altered to reflect heightened concerns for religious authenticity and scientific objectivity.[20]

The ongoing role of scientific medicine in relation to the church's involvement in health care lies at the heart of the next great development in health care, intertwined with the church's missionary vision.[21]

DEVELOPMENT OF SCIENTIFIC MEDICINE AND MEDICAL MISSIONS

Porterfield notes that "the global expansion of Western Christianity in the modern period coincided with the development of scientific medicine and its worldwide preeminence as a resource for human welfare."[22] While preaching/teaching (schools) and print (Bibles and literacy) were the primary means of mission outreach in the modern era, health care was a third component of effective mission. The relationship between scientific medicine and Christian healing, however, has been complex. Missionaries were sent to preach and teach the gospel. A critic of "medical missions" might point out that the term is an oxymoron: medical denotes care of the physical body; the gospel mission is the work of converting people to the Christian faith, sometimes referred to as "saving souls." This dual connotation explains why the start of medical missions faced criticism, and later only reluctant acceptance. Medical missions were not recognized as a legitimate dimension of missions until after 1860. What changed the outlook was the "discovery" that a medical missionary could sometimes gain access to a region or culture that was otherwise closed to priest or pastor.

Presbyterian-ordained medical doctor Peter Parker left New York for Canton, China, in 1834, for a missionary appointment under the Medical Missionary Society. He was charged to subordinate his medical skills and practice to his superior task of teaching the Christian religion. This charge

---

[20]Ibid., p. 118.

[21]For a fascinating read that documents the changing face of medical interventions from ancient to modern times, see the case history on treatments of cancer over four thousand years in Siddhartha Mukherjee, *The Emperor of All Maladies: A Biography of Cancer* (New York: Scribner, 2010).

[22]Porterfield, *Healing in the History of Christianity*, p. 141.

gave Parker considerable agony as he became more and more involved in medical and surgical practice. His American board disapproved his increasing medical priority, and in 1840, when Parker took up diplomatic responsibilities, the board stopped his support.[23] Nonetheless, Peter Parker's contributions bore fruit. Associated more widely with other organizations, Parker went on lecture/preaching tours. His stirring address in Edinburgh (July 26, 1841) led to the formation of the Edinburgh Medical Missionary Society (EMMS) in 1849.[24] Its purpose was that of sponsoring young people who wished to study medicine with a view to foreign missionary service. But most missionary societies were not convinced of the validity of this form of ministry until around 1860.

The first brief training program began at Tübingen, Germany, in 1841, to train missionary physicians in a coordinated ministerial-medical curriculum. With only twelve enrolled, and two graduating—who never went to the field—in its first seven years, the program ended. In 1861 a similar program began and flourished in Edinburgh, largely from the impetus of EMMS.[25]

In 1928 a high-profile British mission representative, Thomas Cochrane, carefully crafted the balance between medicine and mission, "The concern for the body is genuine and sincere; so much that the medical missionary will seek to help with utter abandon and without conditions just as if the healing of the body were an end in itself. But the soul is more precious than the body, and the soul is the supreme concern."[26] Already in 1838, at the beginning of the medical mission enterprise, a purpose statement says,

"HEAL THE SICK" is our motto, constituting alike the injunction under which we act, and the object at which we aim, and which, with the blessing

---

[23]Ibid., pp. 142-43.
[24]Christoffer H. Grundmann, *Sent to Heal! Emergence and Development of Medical Missions* (Lanham, Md.: University Press of America, 2005), pp. 96-97. Grundmann's book is the definitive study of the history and challenges of medical missions. The English publication is the core of his original work, written as a doctoral dissertation and published in German in 1992, filling a gap in studies of mission history. EMMS, with numerous mutations, continues into the present, merging with Emmanuel Hospital Organization (U.K.) into the new Emmanuel Health Care. But the training program as such has long ceased and EHC now operates only the 125-bed hospital in Nazareth, Israel (ibid., pp. 99-100).
[25]Ibid., pp. 95-96.
[26]Ibid., p. xii.

of God, we hope to accomplish, by means of scientific practice, in the exercise of an unbought and untiring kindness.[27]

While this original statement is clear, yet as late as 1947 missiologist Walter Holsten says, "The term 'missionary doctor' places two great realities in relationship to each other. . . . However, what is the relationship between them? Can anyone tell me what a 'missionary doctor' is?"[28] While German mission leaders at their fifth continental conference in 1880 wished to avoid use of the term *medical missions*, the prevailing British and American usage won out.[29]

A second stage to the wide acceptance of medical missions was the discovery that only women could serve other women in many traditional cultures, especially in Muslim and Hindu societies. American women thus established missionary societies to send women ("woman's work for women") to medical school and nurses training and then deployed them to African and Asian countries.

As scientific medicine was introduced into traditional cultures, a critical issue developed: How do missionaries, and especially medical doctors, value the traditional healing practices of the cultures in which they serve? Protestant missionaries usually took a condescending attitude toward such "superstitious" practices, and part of the vision of medical missions was to root out these superstitions and introduce the superior scientific knowledge of the West. However, even the natives who converted to Christianity would often revert to traditional healing practices. "Witch doctors" were readily accessible and these practices made more sense to them than medicine did.

Yet medical missions have had a long and successful track record. Christian churches over the last two centuries have invested an incredible amount of time and money in medical missions. Millions of dollars were invested in China in the late nineteenth and early twentieth centuries.

---

[27]Ibid., p. xiii.

[28]Ibid., p. 1. The term appears to have its origin in correspondence between missionaries of the Danish-Halle or Tranquebar Mission (Southeast India) in 1773 (ibid., pp. 1-2). Prior to that time Jesuit and Franciscan mission doctors were simply called missionaries, who served medical needs. Grundmann narrates the considerable controversy surrounding this term and the notions behind it. Some argued for one role or the other, but not a conflating of the two into one mission, pp. 7-11.

[29]Ibid., pp. 6-7.

Western mission agencies in 1887 "supported forty-one American and thirty-three British medical missionaries in China." American foundations invested heavily in scientific philanthropy: "wealthy Americans—Rockefeller, Ford, Carnegie—. . . understood the dissemination of scientific practice throughout the world as an extension of Protestant missionary strategy."[30]

George Dowkontt (1853-1909), of Polish descent, came to the United States in 1879 from his post as assistant director of the U.K. Liverpool Medical Mission to head up medical mission training in Philadelphia. Then in cooperation with Dwight L. Moody he began similar work in Chicago and later in New York City. His work awakened Seventh-day Adventist Dr. John Harvey Kellogg to support medical missions. J. H. Kellogg began a unique sanitarium (not sanatorium) in Battle Creek, Michigan, constructing a medical curriculum with healthful practices (i.e., preventive medicine) at the center. He developed a series of training programs for "so-called 'Health Missionaries.'" A most skillful surgeon and inventor also, he made a significant contribution to medical missions, delivering around five thousand addresses and performing twenty-two thousand surgeries, never for his own gain but for charitable causes. He and George Dowkonnt together exerted considerable influence in the American Medical Missionary Society (AMMS) in Chicago. With Dowkonnt's untimely death in 1909, and Kellogg's being "disfellowshiped" earlier by the Seventh-day Adventist General Conference over doctrine, Kellogg lost interest in medical missions.[31]

Medical missions nonetheless were understood as a gateway for people to come to Christian faith. A statement from the AMMS in 1883 regarded medical missions as an effective means to evangelize the world. The method, quite pragmatic and deriving from Christ and the apostles, economizes time and funds. "Medical missions can do the most work in the shortest time, because they are the best introducers of the gospel."[32]

---

[30]Porterfield, *Healing in the History of Christianity*, pp. 155-56.

[31]Grundmann, *Sent to Heal*, pp. 115-20. Apparently Kellogg then joined his brother to develop production of healthy food for the next thirty-four years of his life (e.g., Kellogg's cereals). It is sad that mission people who most excelled in medicine, such as Peter Parker and John Harvey Kellogg, experienced conflict with their supporting boards, which ruptured their relationship to the board and to their calling as well (ibid., p. 206).

[32]Ibid., p. 112.

Grundmann describes the theological rationale for medical missions: (1) God's caring love fuels the compassionate witness of medical missions; (2) medical missions function as a health care agency for mission personnel—often sorely needed; and (3) the spiritual empowerment for medical missions is the imitation of Christ (*imitatio Christi*)."[33]

David Livingstone and Albert Schweitzer, African medical missionary icons, inspired many other doctors and nurses to make medical missions and health care their life vocations. Edward Bliss (1865-1960), an outstanding American missionary doctor in China, adopted Livingstone's tomb epitaph as his motto: "'I am a missionary heart and soul. God had an only Son, and He was a missionary and physician.' A poor, poor imitation of Him I am, or hope to be. In this service I hope to live; in it I wish to die."[34]

Schweitzer's life commitment to Jesus' servant ethic shines. Trained with doctorates in three fields (New Testament, music and medicine), Schweitzer's famous *Quest for the Historical Jesus* paved the way for him to understand Jesus existentially, with Jesus' ethic of service unto death the ideal that inspired his life work as a medical missionary.[35] Schweitzer identified with the native peoples in their bearing much pain from disease and impoverished living conditions. He spoke of their common membership in the "fellowship of pain," evoking Paul's view that as suffering humans we share in Jesus' sufferings (Phil 3:10; Col 1:24). He devoted his life to overcome the enemies to human well-being: pain from illness and anguish of spirit. At the same time, he did not value the culture's traditional healing practices but rather scorned them, sometimes telling them to do those things also (cloaked humor) as a way of maintaining rela-

---

[33]Ibid., pp. 207-15.

[34]Edward Bliss Jr., *Beyond the Stone Arches: An American Missionary Doctor in China, 1892-1932* (New York: Wiley, 2001), p. 131, partially cited in Porterfield, *Healing in the History of Christianity*, p. 153. The fuller quotation appears in Grundmann, *Sent to Heal*, p. 8.

[35]Albert Schweitzer, *The Quest of the Historical Jesus* (New York: Macmillan, 1910). The book exposes the failure of the scholarly efforts of the previous 150 years (1750-1900) to find *the* historical Jesus. The widely cited ending to his book helps us understand his life mission in Africa: "He comes to us as One unknown, without a name, as of old, by the lake-side. . . . He says the same words, 'Follow thou me!,' and sets us to those tasks which he has to fulfill for our time. . . . He will reveal Himself in the toils, the conflicts, the sufferings which they shall pass through in His fellowship, and, as an ineffable mystery, they shall learn in their own experience Who He is" (ibid., p. 403; cited in Porterfield, *Healing in the History of Christianity*, p. 148, however, with a different translation).

tionship. But Schweitzer spared no words in condemning the harm and pain caused by colonial rule.[36]

The Christian Medical (and Dental) Associations, originating at Wheaton College, combine mission with medical and dental care. Their mission statement is: "Changing Hearts in Healthcare." Their website describes their vocational commitment:

> The Cross-cultural work breaks down barriers that would otherwise obstruct the Gospel from reaching many around the world, and changes lives forever, both of the person who gives and the person who receives. Our international efforts reach out to those who rarely, if ever, have access to medical or dental health services, and we partner with national organizations to provide educational training so that local healthcare providers can deliver improved care after a team leaves. We often partner with organizations that seek to meet emotional and spiritual needs as well, offering hope that can be found only at the foot of the cross.

While "medical missions" was a driving mission force in Protestant churches, the Roman Catholic Church developed analogous initiatives in the last quarter of the nineteenth century in Francophone Africa, under the leadership of Charles Martial Allemand Lavigerie (1825-1892; became a cardinal in 1882). With training in church history (Sorbonne) forming his moral convictions, he saw "the significance of medical missionary work as a matter of principle rather than a mere tactical strategy." Hence he proposed a completely new approach to missions in his *Mémoir secret*, submitted to Pope Pius IX, January 2, 1878. Thus began the special training that led to the order of the White Fathers, who were trained to be good Christians with thorough training also "in the art of medicine." He said the doctor as missionary would receive "honor and influence" and thus with medical skill be able to dispel the superstitions of the peoples and free them from suffering. He further utilized an indigenous principle, training selected North Africans to take up the medical vocation in central Africa. He developed also a group of "medical catechists" as part of their university education.[37]

In the twentieth century the "face of medical missions changed consid-

---

[36]Cf. Porterfield, *Healing in the History of Christianity*, pp. 121, 147-48.
[37]Grundmann, *Sent to Heal*, pp. 121-23. An outstanding catechist was Adrian Atiman (1864/66-1956) who worked in Tanzania.

erably" with "increasing reliance on indigenous leadership" as well as female specialists, and the "increasingly complicated political worlds that medical missionaries" encounter. Further,

> the medical work sponsored by Christians has become more centralized. Many Christian churches, groups, and individuals support such global agencies as Caritas International Medical Mission Board and Catholic Relief Services of the Roman Catholic Church, the Church World service, which involves thirty Protestant and Orthodox churches, the Evangelical Foreign Missions Association, the American Friends Service Committee, Lutheran World Relief, the Mennonite Central Committee, and the Seventh-day Adventist World Service.[38]

This citation of prominent agencies devoted to helping and healing in areas of need and situations of crisis is not comprehensive. Smaller denominational mission organizations, hundreds of them, plus large interdenominational or nondenominational organizations, from "Save the [Starving] Children" to the Bill and Melinda Gates Foundation, are actively involved in improving health care overseas.

In the historical development of Mennonite missions, health care blended with mission. Since Anabaptist-Mennonite thought and praxis does not dichotomize gospel from ethics, health care functioned integrally to mission.[39] Also by the time Mennonites (in their several denominations) began establishing missions, especially from the 1890s on, the century's earlier debate was settled: medical missions were broadly affirmed. The ideal mission for Mennonite missions was evangelization, education, medicine (including various forms of medical training), and industrial and agricultural development. See appendix one for history on Mennonites and related groups in mission and health care.

---

[38]Porterfield, *Healing in the History of Christianity*, p. 158.
[39]Nonetheless, within the various mission boards differences of opinion and tensions emerged in the discussions of financial support for the larger medical programs.

9

❖

Disability, God's Two Hands of Love

INTERNAL CARE, EXTERNAL WITNESS

*Disabled people are . . . living icons of the crucified Son. They reveal the
mysterious beauty of the One who emptied himself for our sake and made
himself obedient unto death. They show us over and above all appear-
ances that the ultimate foundation of human existence is Jesus Christ. It
is said justifiably . . . that disabled people are humanity's privileged witnesses. They can teach everyone about the love that saves us; they can
become heralds of a new world, no longer dominated by force, violence,
and aggression, but by love, solidarity, and acceptance—a new world
transfigured by the light of Christ, the Son of God, who became in-
carnate, who was crucified, and rose for us.*

Pope John Paul II

The epigraph frames the perspective and concern of this chapter. In the
late 1980s David Barrett pointed out that we might analyze the church's
mission in the world against numerous criteria of concern, ecosystems, a
country's dependence on tourism for economic survival and so forth. A
most important consideration, however, is the reality of megapoverty, ur-
banization and the disabled in this world. From this angle of analysis, he
says (writing in 1987):

> Our world contains 1.6 billion disabled persons, 80 percent in developing
> countries, a third being children, mostly among the absolutely poor in
> Africa, Asia, and Latin America. It also contains 13 million people with
> leprosy, 21 million totally blind persons, 48 million psychotics with severe
> mental disorders, 85 million severely handicapped children, 205 million

partially handicapped children, 450 million deaf persons—of whom 320 million are partially deaf—and 950 million psycho-neurotics.[1]

Barrett says there is no way we can deal adequately with the topic of mission without addressing the needs of those with disabilities. The biblical concept of shalom (Hebrew word for peace) is much related to conditions of justice and economic well-being (see chap. 6). In most literature on shalom the plight of those with disabilities has been overlooked. We need to ask clearly and sharply what shalom means for those with disabilities, whether the disability is physical, mental or emotional. The term *disability* denotes a wide range of circumstances, some in which people function fairly well in society and some with profound learning disorders that need special care and cannot be mainstreamed into societal living.[2]

Regardless of the degree of disability, we should not view the disabled only as *recipients* of the church's concern and ministry. Living with disability, Michael Schwartzentruber reminds us that only as we put the ministry of Jesus Christ in the context of disabilities can we adequately grasp it as good news.[3] Only when we begin to acknowledge and understand our own vulnerability, our pain and even our anger, will we be able to claim the gospel as grace and healing for our own lives. The realistic view of human weakness described in chapter two enables us to identify with the struggle to live that marks the daily life of many with disabilities. Then also we will experience anew the enabling grace of a compassionate God.

This topic is central in conceptualizing the church's mission (see chap. 8). The quality of the church's life and mission is known by its response to the weak, the disabled and the poor in its midst—true in both the Old and

---

[1]David Barrett, "Getting Ready for Mission in the 1990's: What Should We Be Doing to Prepare?" *Missiology: An International Review* 15, no. 1 (January 1987), p. 4.

[2]I use the term *disabled* because recent literature on this topic uses *disability* instead of earlier preferred terms such as *physically* or *mentally challenged*. Since 1996 the scholarly *Journal of Religion, Disability and Health* has addressed a wide range of issues on disability; it regularly uses that term. Syracuse University Press has also begun a new series, Critical Perspectives on Disability, with the first volume a comprehensive study on developments in mental health care as a result of the service of conscientious objectors to war during and after World War II: Steven J. Taylor, *Acts of Conscience: World War II, Mental Institutions, and Religious Objectors*, Critical Perspectives on Disability (Syracuse, N.Y.: Syracuse University Press, 2009).

[3]Michael Schwartzentruber, "The Disabled Church," *Gospel Herald*, March 10, 1988, p. 162. In chap. 3 I pointed out that Jesus' healings are often of those with some degree of disability.

New Testaments. The authenticity of the church's life and mission is evident as church members relate to disabled persons, acknowledging their own weakness, disability and poverty. In these two complementary emphases we discern God's two arms of love: the internal soul of the church and its external witness, both flowing from the same divine compassion.[4] Herein we discover afresh the meaning of Paul's profound testimony: God's strength is made perfect through and in our human weakness.

As described in chapter eight, many mission societies conceptualized the gospel as not only verbal witness but also as a benevolent arm that expressed itself in hospital care of those with physical needs, including disability. The mission response to health care needs demonstrates the two arms of love.[5] The interrelationship of mission word and caring deed requires ongoing discernment within denominations and their congregations. The New Testament books of 1 John and James emphasize the necessity of both arms of love: clear witness to what we believe about Jesus Christ, and expression of that belief in a practicing love that responds to those in need, be it economic or physical. God loves and cares for us in our suffering, in the limitations of our humanity. The ethic and practices of the faith community must reflect the same.

Following, I identify four essential streams of emphasis that require us to hold together external witness and internal care, recognizing these are God's two arms of love.

1. Throughout the Old Testament a recurring motif is the injunction to care for the poor, the widows, the orphans and the alien residents, because such care expresses the justice and love of the Lord God, who redeemed the people of Israel from bondage in Egypt. In the Covenant Code that follows the Ten Commandments in Exodus 20 this specific injunction to show kindness to and care for the needy members of the community punctuates the case laws just as the rising and the setting of the sun punctuate

---

[4]Some readers will recognize the imagery of God's two hands as echoing Martin Luther—used here quite differently than its use with him. Luther employed the imagery to describe God's contrasting means of working through the church and the state. The church lives the love ethic; the state executes God's wrath.

[5]The Mennonite Board of Missions (now Mennonite Mission Network), for example, beginning with its founders, included both the external witness of word *and* internal caring in establishing hospitals (see James Juhnke, *Vision, Doctrine, War: Mennonite Identity and Organization in America 1890-1930* [Scottdale, Penn.: Herald Press, 1989], pp. 139-56). See appendix 1 for the history of Mennonite and related churches in mission and health care.

the markings of time. The practice of this injunction within Israel was the very foundation of their community's expression of justice (see chap. 6). Sample texts occur in Exodus 22:21-27 and Deuteronomy 16:18-20. Justice is intrinsically related to care for the stranger, the widow, the poor, the alien and the oppressed. Care for those with special needs in the community is a basic form of social justice. The story of lame Mephibosheth (2 Sam 4:4; 9; 19:24-30), whom David invites to eat from his table for life, illustrates special kindness in keeping with these biblical themes of mercy and justice.

2. When Jesus came into Galilee proclaiming the gospel of the kingdom of God, it appears that his mission was primarily that of *word:* proclaiming that the time is fulfilled, the kingdom is at hand, repent and believe the gospel (Mk 1:15). But in the gospel narratives Jesus' deeds of healing the disabled in body and spirit are pervasive, even though he clearly says that his mission is to preach and teach (Mk 1:38). The first half of Mark shows Jesus spending most of his time responding to human need through healings, exorcisms and feeding the hungry. It is similar in Matthew and Luke, and to a lesser extent in John (see Jn 5–6; 9; 11).

Some commentators regard Jesus' healing ministry as peripheral to the gospel, if not an outright interruption. It was not part of Jesus' real ministry: calling people into the reign of God. But most commentators regard the manner of Jesus' proclamation as significant: the kingdom of God was proclaimed precisely in the deeds of healing, liberating those possessed by unclean spirits, opening the eyes of the blind and healing the outcast lepers (fulfilling the messianic hope of Is 35; 61:1-2). Jesus' compassionate caring is neither a detour nor an adjunct to the witness of the word; it fundamentally expresses the good news of the gospel of peace. Matthew 9:35; 10:1; and Luke 9:2; 10:9 are crystal clear that curing the sick is essential to the disciples' proclamation of the kingdom of God come near. Healing is intrinsic to Jesus'—and our—gospel mission.[6]

Current trends emphasize that Jesus' shalom gospel liberates from economic and political injustice. While this is also true, the accent in the Gospels falls on good news for the disabled, whether in body, mind or spirit.

---

[6]Scot McKnight emphasizes the central thread of the kingdom of God in Jesus' mission, making a similar point: "The mission of Jesus is healing justice, the ending of disease, dislocation, and oppression," in *A Community Called Atonement* (Nashville: Abingdon, 2007), p. 13.

For this reason the interrelationship between the mission of the church and our experience of vulnerability and response to disability express the heart of God's gospel in and through Jesus Christ and his disciples.

3. This fundamental unity, expressed in God's two arms of love, both word and deed, turns up in the Pauline letters. We normally think of Paul as the great missionary apostle, the apostle to the Gentiles, the one who risked his life for the proclamation of the good news to all people. This is true indeed, but Paul's proclaiming the gospel, which many Gentiles accepted, included also God's arm of love in healing (Acts 14:8-10; 16:16-18; 19:11-20; cf. Acts 20:9-12) and mutual caring for one another (see chap. 7). In speaking about charismatic or spiritual gifts, Paul includes the gift of healing (1 Cor 12:9, 28). When Paul visited the three pillar apostles in Jerusalem, he learned nothing new about the nature of the gospel to the Gentiles, except he agreed with them that "he should remember the poor" (Gal 2:10). Much of Paul's missionary energy was expended on raising funds throughout the Gentile churches to care for the physical needs of brothers and sisters in Jerusalem.

The proclamation of the word to the Gentiles and the ministry of monetary relief to the Jewish Christians are two sides of the same gospel coin. On this point the gospel of Jesus Christ cannot be dichotomized; nor can one part be carried forward authentically without the other part. The two go hand in hand; they are indeed two arms of the same loving compassionate God.

4. John's test for authentic discipleship applies specifically to this dimension of care within the Christian community: "By this everyone will know that you are my disciples, if you have love for one another" (Jn 13:34). In John's epistles the matter is put forthrightly: we cannot say that we belong to God if we do not care for the needs of Christian brothers and sisters (1 Jn 3:16-18).

These two arms of external witness and internal care for one another provide the biblical foundation for our churches to be accessible to all as intrinsic to our mission.

SEEING WITH NEW EYES: BEAUTY AND GRACE IN DISABILITY

Jesus had compassion for those socially marginalized by physical illness and disability (Mk 2:1-8; Jn 5:1-12; 9:1-20). Two of the people in these chapters were paraplegic (we no longer use the term *paralytic*). Those who suffer from this disability lack feeling in their lower body and are especially vulnerable to illnesses because detection is difficult. Jesus took initiative to connect with the disabled in John (in the Mark 2 passage friends bring the man to Jesus) in order to heal and restore them to social functioning in their communities.[7] This challenges us in our attitudes and practices of life. The story in John 5 describes a chronic illness and the neglect and exploitation of the suffering one.

While we may not have the power that Jesus had to heal instantly, we can become a healing presence by accommodating to their needs, and in our own weaknesses identifying with them in their infirmities.

In university and seminary education we should accommodate those with mobile or sensory disabilities, trying to provide help and resources to enable them to be full participants in the learning experience.[8] Important also is their enriching the learning process by presenting their perspectives of (biblical) interpretation. When our bothers and sisters in the faith are hospitalized or in nursing homes, do we commit to visit and include them socially as much as is possible? The challenge before us is willingness to experience "vulnerable communion," a term Reynolds unpacks in seven chapters: developing a theology of disability, which has impact on communal boundaries that overcome "the cult of normalcy" and enable us to dwell together; a rethinking of what we mean by "able bodies" so that we own our illusion of control and denial of vulnerability; recovering disability that opens us to the other and to vulnerability; our understanding of divine love and how it bears upon creation; our worthiness of God's love; and togetherness in hospitality within the faith community. Vulnerable communion restores us to one another and to God.[9]

The writings and DVDs of Jean Vanier, who lives among the disabled in L'Arche communities, inspire us.[10] They also lift the veil from our eyes

---

[7]See the contributions by John Pilch in the bibliography. These emphasize the restoration to community life as an important component of Jesus' healing mission. Similarly, see Hector Avalos, Sarah J. Melcher and Jeremy Schipper, eds., *This Abled Body: Rethinking Disabilities in Biblical Studies* (Atlanta: Society of Biblical Literature, 2007); and Sharon V. Betcher, *Spirit and the Politics of Disablement* (Minneapolis: Fortress, 2007).

[8]Many of us who have taught in these settings have not done as well as we might have.

[9]Thomas E. Reynolds, *Vulnerable Communion: A Theology of Disability and Hospitality* (Grand Rapids: Brazos Press, 2008).

[10]For introduction to numerous L'Arche communities and the challenges they present, see the

to see beauty in these persons. They love and appreciate personal relationships, desire connectedness and want others to value their personal worth. Mark Bredin, who has provided care and assistance for children with severe disability, came to see and write about true beauty in the disabled.[11] Bredin says that by relating to those with disability (whether learning, physically or emotionally disabled) we discover a new dimension of God's grace. Drawing on Jürgen Moltmann, Bredin remarks that the false notions of our modern culture—the image of the ideal body—prevent us from seeing the beauty in those disabled and disfigured.[12] We need an attitudinal change. By taking up the servant stance exemplified by Jesus, and committing ourselves to seek shalom (well-being) for all, we will personally experience transformation and transformed relationships with the disabled. We will seek community for and with them. Such relationships challenge our competitive approach to life and open up deeper and more satisfying life experiences. By providing community for the disabled we learn what interdependence is and perceive our own poverty of spirit. Our poverty and loneliness are exposed; we identify with Jesus' spirit of compassion that heals human brokenness. Henri Nouwen sees the disabled as a gift of community; they are the means of kingdom blessing to us:

> More than ever, I believe in the gift of handicapped people to create . . . community. Their weakness is God's strength; their dependence is God's invitation to create bonds of love and support; their poverty is one of God's ways to bring us the blessings of the Kingdom.[13]

Compassion for the disabled will mean praying for and anointing the sick (Jas 5:13-18) and sustaining relationships of love and care. We will value *gentleness* and *interdependence* in our relationship with the disabled, as John McGee has taught us.[14] Health care will mean not only insurance coverage or mutual aid, both extremely important, but also inclusion of the

---

multiauthored book *The Challenge of L'Arche* (Minneapolis: Winston Press, 1981).

[11] Mark Bredin, *True Beauty: Finding Grace in Disabilities*, Grove Spirituality Series (Cambridge: Grove Books, 2007).

[12] Ibid., p. 4. Stanley Hauerwas and Jean Vanier also speak to this topic in *Living Gently in a Violent World: The Prophetic Witness of Weakness* (Downers Grove, Ill.: InterVarsity Press, 2008).

[13] Henri Nouwen, "The Gulf Between East and West," *New Oxford Review*, May 1994, p. 16.

[14] John J. McGee and Frank J. Menolascino, *Beyond Gentle Teaching: A Nonaversive Approach to Helping Those in Need* (New York: Plenum Press, 1991). See also the groundbreaking work of Wolf Wolfensberger on understanding of and care for mentally ill persons ("The Theological Voice of Wolf Wolfensberger," *Journal of Religion, Disability & Health* 4, nos. 2-3 [2001]: 149-57).

sick and disabled into our community life, as much as possible. Accessibility issues will be addressed and cared for. We will do whatever it takes to put them "at the table" of fellowship, communion and grace, for they will enable us all to experience a fuller dimension of God's grace and the community it generates.

Only as we grasp this perspective will we own our vulnerability and brokenness. Our eyes will see the disabled in a new light, in the light of God, Jesus and the Spirit. The wholeness of the gospel of peace will include the disabled as an intrinsic part of our church communities. The families of those with disabilities have special needs in pastoral care.[15] Only as professional health teams and congregations join hands in responding to disability needs will the family members receive adequate care for their pain and hurt. Congregations need to see supportive care for the disabled and their families as part of their local mission.[16] Praying and weeping, praising and laughing will bind together those who give and receive care. Distinctions between the two will blur as all of God's children know themselves to be both disabled and enabled by the gift of God's Spirit.

As disabled Michael Schwartzentruber concludes his article:

> In the image of the crucified Christ, we witness God's identification with and participation in the weakness and vulnerability of human existence. But more than that, we also *experience* this identification and participation. For we are not just *adam*, *nephesh*, and *basar*. We possess . . . *ruah*, the gift of God's Spirit. With it comes the power to accept and work within our limitations and thereby in a sense overcome them. *Ruah* is the power of God to transform our spiritual brokenness into spiritual wholeness, our weakness into strength, our disability into ability.[17]

---

[15]See here the story of a mother caring for her disabled son and the theological reflection accompanying her experience: Frances Young, *Face to Face: A Narrative Essay in the Theology of Suffering* (Edinburgh: T & T Clark, 1990). Stanley Hauerwas narrates the great difficulty of maintaining spousal relation with one suffering mental disability in his *Hannah's Child: A Theologian's Memoir* (Grand Rapids: Eerdmans, 2010), pp. 123-50.

[16]See Dean A. Preheim-Bartel et al., *Supportive Care in the Congregation: Providing a Congregational Network of Care for Persons with Significant Disabilities*, rev. ed. (Harrisonburg, Va.: Mennonite Publishing, 2011); Erik W. Carter, *Including People with Disabilities in Faith Communities: A Guide for Service Providers, Families, and Congregations* (Baltimore, Md.: Paul H. Brookes, 2007); Amos Yong, *The Bible, Disability and the Church: A New Vision of the People of God* (Grand Rapids: Eerdmans, 2011).

[17]Schwartzentruber, "Disabled Church," p. 163.

All of us are the disabled church. And as such, we are in God's image. We are the brokenness in the world, with which God, through Christ crucified, has chosen to identify. But as the disabled church we are *enabled* and *gifted* through the Holy Spirit to be representatives of God's transforming and creative power and presence in the world for all people, with whatever challenging situation we face.

COMMITTING TO ACCESS FOR THE DISABLED

As we set goals for our churches and schools we do well to include in our thinking the many disabled people in our world and ask what provisions we are making for them in these goals. What impact will this consideration have on our goals in light of the biblical theology in which external witness and internal care are part of the same gospel coin? As Stanley Hauerwas contends, it is not enough to develop a theory about corporate societal responsibility for the disabled (à la Martha Nussbaum), but that which makes Christian service different is opening our lives to be in living relationships with them and to learn from them, as Jean Vanier has done in the L'Arche communities.[18]

Setting goals that include the disabled in the community may mean increased giving so that the percentage of income allocated to charity moves from an average of 5 percent to 10 percent or more of total income. In view of David Barrett's data that over one-fourth of the world's population consists of people with disabilities, what does this mean for our church's mission in the world? If we are ambassadors of the whole gospel, it will mean holistic care for all, with our community life incorporating the disabled, those easily marginalized by the success values of our Western society.

It also means that our vision for church growth dare not be triumphal. If we are to minister to the needs of the whole person we will include the disabled. This may help us understand better the New Testament call to participate in the sufferings of Christ (Phil 3:10; Col 1:24). We will need to heed the cry of the one-fourth of the world's

---

[18]Hauerwas and Vanier, *Living Gently*, pp. 21-58. See also Hauerwas's article, "The Politics of Gentleness: Abled and Disabled," *Christian Century*, December 2, 2008, pp. 28-32, and the review of three recent books on disability in Brian Volck, "Toward a Theology of Disability," *Christian Century*, December 2, 2008, pp. 32-34.

population, "if you will, you are able to help me to wholeness." This health care task is no less a mission of the church than is the support of pastors and overseas missionaries.

Once our hearts are touched and our minds committed, then we will formulate goals for health care both in the congregation's ministry and in our society's professional care. We will commit ourselves to inclusive facilities and to inclusive relationships. We will need to think also how we respond to the varied cultural needs that will be an increasing part of the population of our health care facilities. Our church services will include prayers for healing, not that physical disabilities will miraculously disappear (though God sometimes surprises us with just such a sign of his grace and power), but to enable us in our disabilities to find God's caring presence and power to heal our brokenness. We will pray that God will empower us in our weaknesses, our vulnerability and compromised health circumstances.

In developing strategies for church colleges and universities we must include preparing students to serve in provider centers for the disabled. This planning will encourage higher educational institutions to remember two important virtues in our Christian heritage: humility and service. It will affect the philosophy behind career counseling, including possibly college education for the disabled, about which Elissa Cooper passionately writes.[19] It will produce more Certified Nursing Assistants who see this vocation as opportunity for important Christian service. It will develop a stronger link between Christian service and schools' nursing and pre-medical professional health care training.

After my dad's death I remember the struggle that we as a family went through to know how to provide adequate health care for my brother, Clifford, whose learning ability held him at fifth grade. With Indian Creek Homes having recently begun (the late 1960s), we had a place for

---

[19]Elissa Cooper, "Why Not College for the Disabled?" *Christianity Today*, November 2010, pp. 17-19. The subtitle is "New Faith-Based School Opens Doors for Young Adults with Intellectual Disabilities," which is about Union Grove, Wisconsin. She quotes Debra Hart, a Boston-based educational coordinator, who identifies three types of programs available for those with disability: the "inclusive individual support model," with peers who provide tutorial support; the "hybrid model," where students with disability take classes on life skills, attending these classes with other students; and a "substantially separate model," where students with disability learn vocational and social skills appropriate to their capabilities and needs (ibid., p. 18). Union Grove represents the third model.

him. It was and is church-sponsored, an expression of the caring love of God's people.[20] Clifford had a special, valued way of being. He frequently gave his intuitive analysis that "some people aren't what they think they are." "God looks on the heart."

Learning from my brother I propose that the existence and work of residences for the disabled remind our society, "You are not what you think you are." Here, where the realities of life are reduced to basic perspectives, with limitations, vulnerability, pain and tears as well as residents' care-free living, love and laughter, we learn who we really are in our corporate humanity. Moreover, as happens when the church embraces its mission holistically, we know through the presence of the empowering Spirit that God is strangely in our midst, as compassionate companion in our suffering and hope.

---

[20]Indian Creek Homes is administered by Indian Creek Foundation, Souderton, Pennsylvania. Such disability organizations across the U.S. are "sponsored" in a coordinating supervisory role by Mennonite Health Services Alliance in Goshen, Indiana. (See appendix 1.)

PART THREE

Toward
New Paradigms

10

❖

Health Care Reform

EVALUATION AND PROSPECTS

There is near universal agreement among thoughtful leaders that [health care] reform is necessary. Our country is on an unsustainable path of spending larger portions of the nations' productivity and wealth on health care [than other countries]. . . . As Christians, we are guided to love our neighbor as ourselves and to care for those unable to care for themselves. So, the question is not whether health care and health care financing should be available to all, but rather how can we best arrange the talents God provides to accomplish our objective.

Terrie E. Troxel,
"Health Care Reform: Don't Trust It to the Angels"

People who call the U.S. system "the best in the world" must not know that we spend 40% more per capita (for hospitals, doctors, medications, and supplies) than any other nation, but are not 40% healthier, as measured by length of life, deaths of newborns, or any other standard yardstick. Yes, some people in every nation have bad experiences; there is no miraculously perfect system of assuring that everyone gets the care he or she needs, when it's needed, with no errors and no interpersonal tension.

Kristine M. Gebbie,
"Health Care Reform: Get Everyone In!"

INTRODUCTORY CONCEPTS

What do we mean by *health care*? We think of doctors, nurses, psychiatrists, hospitals and clinics, but its range is broader, for it includes pharmacists as well as companies researching new drugs, social workers, physical therapists, nursing and retirement centers, and hospice. Do we think also of chaplains and pastors as part of the healing ministries? We must not overlook the spiritual dimension of holistic health care. Health care also includes prevention: education and practices that promote healthy lifestyles that avoid habits and practices that cause illness. Genetic factors are important as well.

Health care also includes the manufacturing and sales of numerous medical devices, from eyeglasses to hearing aids, pacemaker/defibrillators and many more technological devices. Surgeries of all kinds, with greater or lesser degrees of success, abound in modern health care. Through numerous interventions directed usually to individuals, but sometimes to populations, as in vaccines, hospitals and related care centers, the prevailing goal of health care is to restore to health and maximize wellness.

Health education includes knowledge of how to maximize the benefits of today's health care resources. Its goal is to help consumers of health care detect early signs of illness and seek appropriate treatment by utilizing the best current professional understandings and resources. Even with advanced medical knowledge and technology, a degree of educated guessing, however, is often necessary. Numerous tests utilizing technology, however, reduce guesswork and make more accurate diagnoses. But technology is not to be used simply because it's available or to increase salaries for health care providers.

The financing of health care and its costs differs greatly from country to country. Most Western countries, with the exception of the United States, finance their health care systems through a single-payer method. The federal government is usually that single payer, and taxes are paid by all citizens to finance the health care system. This is similar to the U.S. Social Security tax, which finances Medicare. The U.S. financing of Medicaid, however, is shared between states and federal government. Universal health care access means all citizens and residents within a country have equal access to health care, at least in principle. However, universal health care and single-payer financing are not coordinates. Japan, for example, has universal health care access but nearly 3,500 insurance companies, far more than any other country. However, its federal government has standardized fees for all health services.

Unfortunately, in the United States today *health care* has narrowed down to "Obamacare," *yes* (with hope) or *no* (with derision), with either response predicting dire fiscal consequences "if not done." This is unfortunate. Health care means so much more than its present economic-political captivity. In its historical, theological and moral context the prophetic phrase "with healing in its wings" (Mal 4:2), signifies what health care ought to be, as the topical progression in this book demonstrates. Health care ought to ring hope, gift and gratitude in our hearts and minds, with God and scientific knowledge and skills together a blessing for us all.

ANALYSIS OF HEALTH CARE IN THE UNITED STATES

U.S. health care has many different players in its system of financing and delivery. The system-industry is complex; fixing it is a daunting task.

Why is health care so costly in the United States? The main reason is that the U.S. system includes many players in the health care industry. Further, health insurance is costly because insurance companies, health care management companies and the health care providers receive generous salaries, which for younger doctors help pay off sizeable student debt.[1] Some CEOs seek exorbitant salaries, and some doctors order more tests than necessary. The fiduciary responsibility of health insurance companies creates a disincentive to cover medical expenses if they can be avoided. The complexity of administrating health care combined with the many "players" in the system makes health care costly, tedious and sometimes onerous. Dr. Mary Zennett says,

> I can attest to the impact of managed care and utilization review on practitioners and patients. During the advent of managed care in the 1990s, I've mentioned feeling as if someone had turned up the speed on a treadmill, and none of us—not doctors, patients, nurses, or administrative staff—was

---

[1]Medical school costs are high, resulting in swelling student debt. This has a deleterious effect on the availability of medical professionals, which in turn has impact on access. The American Medical Association and Medical Student Society are lobbying federal agencies to address this problem. For more on this, see www.ama-assn.org/ama/pub/about-ama/our-people/member-groups-sections/medical-student-section/advocacy-policy/medical-student-debt.page?

getting off. The only way to slow down the pace of practice with managed care was to refuse to accept any insurance reimbursement or to leave practice.[2]

Zennett cites evidence to demonstrate how the various players in health care make the system so costly (e.g., suits for malpractice, which in some instances stem from patients' dissatisfaction from the lack of time medical staff give to their needs). Zennett attributes this trend to the overwhelming amount of time required for paperwork to meet all the requirements set by funding parties, and they are many.

The following list, lumping together several categories of third-party payers, visualizes the complexity of the health care system in the United States.

1. consumers (the patients)

2. employers (who provide full or partial health insurance for employees)

3. personnel providers (physicians, nurses and other health care workers)

4. facility providers (hospitals, trauma centers, surgical centers, etc.)

5. third-party players in the system:[3]

   • health care insurance companies
   • brokers who negotiate between the insurance companies and providers
   • managed care companies (HMOs, PPOs; adding complexity and costs)
   • health care researchers: those who develop technology and new drugs
   • numerous companies that sell Part D drug Medicare coverage

6. suppliers of drugs (pharmaceutical companies) and costly media promotion

7. suppliers of medical devices, technology of various sorts, and other equipment—costs growing at an alarming rate

8. attorneys (whose fees are costly)

9. malpractice insurance for protection of hospital and medical personnel

The multiparty payer system generates a huge amount of paperwork for providers. Any given provider has to bill many insurance companies or Medicare or Medicaid. Gebbie speaks of "thousands of different, com-

---

[2]Dr. Mary Zennett, *Health for US All: The Transformation of U.S. Health Care* (Colorado Springs: Third Day Press, 2009), p. 12.

[3]Some minority groups, outside-system players such as the Amish, negotiate directly with hospitals and other providers. Bypassing several levels of market industry, they avoid some of the higher costs.

peting insurance plans" and "up to one hundred different variations on payment schedule, coverage, and billing."[4] For Medicare patients with supplemental insurance, two billings are required. Insurance companies hire employees to determine amounts of reimbursement.

Suppliers of drugs, medical devices and equipment play a major role in the cost of health care, for they negotiate directly with providers or management care companies. Those without insurance often find that a given medical procedure or drug costs more for them than if they had insurance, since Medicare or insurance companies negotiate limits to the cost of a given medical procedure or drug. Attorneys also play a significant role, as do costly consultants and umpires at all levels.

This complexity of the U.S. health care system works against efficiency. Health care costs are inordinately high because each of the different players must make a profit and survive the competition. Hence, the result is the spiraling cost of health insurance and the never-ending processing of which medicines are covered, which insurance company has the lowest premium and which provides the best coverage for one's particular needs. Those with Part D prescription drug coverage need to reassess annually which provider covers their prescribed drugs at the most reasonable cost. This requires juggling the copay cost with the deductible level. Annual reassessment is necessary since the various Part D companies bargain with the pharmaceutical companies and end up in any given year with more or less cost-effective contracts. Consumers need counsel, and this too is another layer of expense in the system, unless done by volunteers. Aren't there any initiatives to simplify such a complex plan? Consumers of U.S. health care generally have difficulty understanding the system and tend to be passive patients. Dr. Glen Miller stresses empowering the patient to understand how to maximize health care benefits and reduce its costs.[5] His analysis, arising from his years of medical service as an M.D. in several countries, is helpful to those of us who are not medical professionals.

From her experience as a primary care provider, Zennett describes the frustration that the complex U.S. health care system causes for providers,

Many health care professionals agree that lack of access to care is among

---

[4]Kristine M. Gebbie, "Health Care Reform: Get Everyone In!" *Word & World* 30 (2010): 99.
[5]Glen E. Miller, *Empowering the Patient: How to Reduce the Cost of Health Care and Improve Its Quality* (Indianapolis: Dog Ear, 2009).

the greatest strains on our health care system today. This includes care for people covered partly or minimally under health insurance. My staff and I spend almost as much time being creative in helping people get the [coverage] care they need as we do treating patients. This is no small statement, as we care for large numbers of patients daily. And we are not alone. I hear stories of health care staff providing free care, markedly reduced care, writing off copayments and insurance deductibles, providing pharmaceutical samples, helping patients apply for patient assistance programs from pharmaceutical companies, or offering patients taxi vouchers just to get home from doctor's visits. Such activities have become an additional and standard part of a health provider's already very busy day.

Here in the United States, with the highest per capita costs on heathcare in the world and where costs are rising exponentially, the World Health Organization ranks the overall quality of our health care system as thirty-seventh.[6]

This WHO ranking of the United States as thirty-seventh dates from 2000. The ranking provoked much debate regarding the "conceptual framework underlying the rankings," that is, the criteria used for measurement. Comparisons were based largely on "the extent to which investments in public health and medical care were contributing to critical social objectives: improving health, reducing health disparities, protecting households from impoverishment due to medical expenses, and providing responsive services that respect the dignity of the patient."[7] The report's data was based on applying "the framework to a quantitative assessment of the performance of 191 national health care systems."[8]

As the counterpoint essays in this chapter epigraph exemplify, philosophies regarding *how* health care reform is best achieved differ. Troxel contends that the House Bill 3200 would add $1 trillion to the federal budget over the next ten years, pushing the country into deeper debt. This would not fulfill the moral goal of love for neighbor.[9] Gebbie, however, says that "the tenfold difference in administrative costs between Medicare and private

[6]Zennett, *Health for US All*, p. 8.
[7]See the article by Christopher J. L. Murray and Julio Frenk, "Ranking 37th—Measuring the Performance of the U.S. Health Care System," in *New England Journal of Medicine* 362 (2010): 98.
[8]Ibid. However this figure is assessed, these authors point out that it is "hard to ignore that in 2006, the United States was number 1 in terms of health care spending per capita but ranked 39th for infant mortality, 43rd for adult male mortality, and 36th for life expectancy" (ibid.).
[9]Terrie E. Troxel, "Health Care Reform: Don't Trust It to the Angels," *Word & World* 30 (2010): 100.

coverage demonstrates potential savings."[10] John Toussaint, founder and president of the innovative ThedaCare Center for Healthcare Value, says:

> Today's health care all too often is plagued with waste, errors, and high costs. As a result, the industry crashes an equivalent of a 747 jet each day, meaning about three hundred people die unnecessarily from medical errors, according to the Institute of Medicine.
>
> These statistics are wholly unacceptable. Yet they are a direct result of disjointed care, where waste is rampant, clear communication is missing, and traditional barriers block staff collaboration. Our patients—and our fellow healthcare providers, who work in this environment each day—deserve better.
>
> The solution isn't only about having electronic health records, more insurance coverage, or more advanced technology. Unless we fix the waste and errors first, all we're doing is developing different ways to pay for and perpetuate a broken system. Patients deserve a cohesive care experience that gets them better, faster and home, sooner, i.e. care that costs less and increases value. Lean healthcare helps us create this unique model. Manufacturers have used lean thinking for decades to achieve steady productivity gains, reduced defects, and improved customer care and employee experiences. Imagine similar results in healthcare![11]

President Obama's first signed bill granted health insurance coverage to 4.1 million more children (the total number of children covered now by the U.S. government is over 11 million). This curbed the percentage of the uninsured, but the rising unemployment, with many losing insurance, offset the gain. In his first speech to Congress, Obama called for further commitment to health care reform, most emphatically that it "should not wait, cannot wait, and will not wait another year." The March 2010 health care reform bill, "Affordable Care Act," marks a crucial turning point. It will likely be modified as political parties seek to resolve the budget di-

---

[10]Kristine M. Gebbie, "Health Care Reform," p. 101.
[11]John Toussaint, "ThedaCare's Lean Approach to Primary Care," *Medical Home News* 2.6, June 2010, p. 1. Available at www.createhealthcarevalue.com/data/blog/ Medical Home News - June 2010.pdf. This comparison to a Jetliner crash every day is one Richard Stearns also uses to help us realize the immense tragedy of children dying from preventable causes related to poverty. Only in that case, it's 100 crashes every day totaling 26,500 people dying (Richard Stearns, *The Hole in Our Gospel* [Nashville: Thomas Nelson, 2009], pp. 106-7). Virtually all these deaths result from lack of or inadequate health care, as Stearns's chapters 10-13 (pp. 114-60) document.

lemmas facing the nation. Special interest groups like American Medical Association, insurance companies and pharmaceutical companies wield power to modify the reform bill to enhance their own "chip" of the health care market. But reform has begun. As more people benefit from the Affordable Care Act the momentum for change will likely increase.

Some states have led the way to enroll all state residents in health care. Massachusetts, during Governor Mitt Romney's leadership, was the first, beginning July 1, 2007. An update article in the November 22, 2010, *Newsweek* reports 93 percent are insured, and costs have not gone up more than expected despite an influx of new patients. In early 2011 Vermont, under Governor Peter Shumlin's leadership, also adopted a similar universal care initiative that "guarantees coverage not linked to employment, and a single system of provider payments and administrative rules," but it will "remain privately owned." This initiative may be a pilot project, on a small scale (625,000 population), for the United States implementation in successive phases of the Affordable Care Act.[12] "In June 2006 San Francisco mayor Gavin Newsom unveiled his proposal to offer a health care plan for all city residents. "Revenue . . . would come from taxpayers, voluntary business contributions, and monthly premiums. The plan was approved the next month."[13] These initiatives, together with the Affordable Care Act and Patients Bill of Rights, bolster hope for greater accessibility in the future.

In a time of economic meltdown, as in 2007-2009, some employers hired employees through temporary employment agencies to avoid the costly benefit of health care insurance. This practice together with rising unemployment increases the number of uninsured. From 2004-2010 the rising cost of health insurance forced a growing number of employers to shift more of the cost to the employee in order for their businesses to be competitive.[14] The employer who has to face the hard decision to terminate

---

[12]Anya Rader Wallack, "Single Payer Ahead—Cost Control and the Evolving Vermont Model," *New England Journal of Medicine* 365, no. 7 (2011): 584. Further detail in the article is informative.

[13]Mary McDonough, *Can a Health Care Market Be Moral? A Catholic Vision* (Washington, D.C.: Georgetown University Press, 2007), p. 209.

[14]The United States' largest employer, Walmart, for all its partly justified criticism, is to be congratulated for affirming (late June 2009) President Obama's efforts to require employers to provide health care insurance to all employees. But Walmart must now practice what it then affirmed. *CBS Evening News* (Oct. 21, 2011; "Walmart trims health care coverage for some")

workers carries a moral burden as well: it means putting employees at risk of losing health insurance. The unemployed also cannot afford health insurance with a high deductible. If they pay the first $5,000, or even $2,500, the policy is of little help; it is not practical for unemployed people or for those with low income. As a result the health care insurance industry is downsized, since more and more of the population goes without insurance. Hospitals are left with unpaid bills. The cost forces some people (with mental illness) to go off the medications necessary for good health, and this creates another societal hazard.

From December 2008 to July 2009 unemployment increased monthly, increasing the number of uninsured. The COBRA provision of the stimulus bill, covering 65 percent of the health insurance cost for companies with over twenty employees, enabled some unemployed persons to continue health insurance. But many could not afford insurance even with COBRA's help. When unemployed, even 35 percent of the health care insurance cost is not affordable.[15] High unemployment continues to persist through 2011, causing both loss of health insurance and many home foreclosures.

In light of U.S. health care costs, more U.S. citizens are traveling to other countries to get less costly health care for specific treatments. Rick Johnson speaks of the growing "flat-world health care" trends, where less costly health care overseas attracts more and more Americans. Since employers often include a "travel budget" in employees' salaries, employees may elect to have surgical procedures done overseas, saving thousands of dollars. A $40,000 knee surgery in the United States could be done in Taiwan for $10,000, for example.[16] Some companies' health insurance

---

announced that Walmart will now deny health insurance for part-time employees (those working less than twenty-four hours weekly) and will raise its already high health insurance premiums 20-50 percent next year. Many employees (e.g., one featured on CBS who earns $9.40 per hour) cannot afford this and will decline insurance, thus increasing the number of the uninsured. See www.reuters.com/article/2011/10/21/us-walmart-idUSTRE79K43Z20111021. Safeway's grocery chain deserves commendation for providing employee incentives to lower their body mass index and encourage weight loss and healthy eating.
[15]In November 2008, NPR reported that two million people lost their health insurance each month over the past several months (i.e., August-October 2008), due to job losses and people not able to pay insurance premiums.
[16]Rick Johnson, "Flat-World Health Care," *HealthLeaders*, January 2009, p. 29. Johnson cites comparative costs from Josef Woodman, "Everybody's Guide to Affordable, World-Class Medical Tourism," in *Patients Beyond Borders* (Chapel Hill, N.C.: Healthy Travel Media, 2008). The article shows the comparative costs for specific interventions such as heart bypass (U.S.: $70,000-$133,000; Singapore: $16,300; Panama: $10,500), knee replacement and so

benefits now include emergency medical attention for their employees' travel. The lower cost of overseas surgeries saves expense and increases profits for the employer and its insurance company as well.

More recent comparative costs among five different countries indicate the U.S. costs are over two to five times higher than in other Western countries. Examples are:[17]

	Britain	Canada	France	Germany	U.S.
M.R.I. scan	$ 187	304	398	632	1,009
Avg. hospital stay	N.A	7,707	4,715	4,718	14,427
*Cataract surgery	1,299	927	3,352	N.A.	14,764
Hip replacement	9,637	10,753	12,629	15,329	34,454
Bypass surgery	13,998	22,212	16,325	27,237	59,770

Hospitals and medical clinics need to assess and evaluate how much of an employee's work time provides value to the patient. Some studies show that of the time taken to admit a patient for surgery only about 30 percent contributes value to the patient. The other time is spent looking for supplies and equipment, asking the patient unnecessary questions, drawing unnecessary blood, or retracing one's steps to pick up something that was forgotten.

---

forth in eight different countries. More and more people are flying overseas for nonemergency procedures. The article cites from the Deloitte Center for Health Solutions "that by 2010 as many as 6 million Americans may travel abroad for care." A professor colleague of mine chooses to have his dental work done when visiting relatives in Argentina. But shopping around in the United States may turn up a similar sharp reduction in costs. A news item in the *AARP Bulletin*, April 2009, tells how Rodney Larson, who needed triple bypass surgery, saved 80 percent cost by going to Galichia Hospital in Wichita, Kansas, in comparison to having it done in his Minnesota home area ($13,200 compared to $80,000).

[17]Philip M. Boffey, "The Money Traps in U.S. Health Care," *New York Times*, January 22, 2012, p. SR 12. Boffey's data source for this is the International Federation of Health Plans. More "procedure" examples are given in the article, as well as other comparative data: length of "waiting" time to see a specialist; breast cancer 5-year survival rates; and asthma hospital admission rates. Among the five countries, the U.S. is second shortest in length of "waiting," first in 5-year cancer survival and highest in hospital admissions for asthma (over seven times more than Canada, 121:16). Boffey says the health reform law could curb total spending, partly by "bundling" payments to hospitals and doctors. Boffey's data source for this latter information is Commonwealth Fund (wait times): Organization for Economic Cooperation and Development.

*A correction appeared online (*New York Times*) January 30, 2012, that the International Federation of Health Plans calculated the cost of U.S. cataract surgery to include "inpatient hospital costs." When performed in outpatient facilities the average is revised to $3,161—quite a difference!

RECAPPING WHY HEALTH CARE REFORM IS ESSENTIAL

However difficult health care reform is for the United States the "what" and "why" factors that make reform essential are:

- Until the March 2010 Affordable Care Act was implemented in September 2010, around 50 million did not have health insurance and received health care only under emergency situations. Beginning in 2014 and by 2016, it is estimated by the nonpartisan Congressional Budget Office, along with the congressional Joint Committee on Taxation, that 32 million of those previously uninsured will be insured. However, this might change in Congress's ongoing deliberations.

- Millions more are underinsured: Medicaid or Medicare does not cover all expenses. Insurance companies, with their high deductibles and copays, also do not cover all expenses. These factors indicate how far the United States is from the universal coverage of most wealthy Western nations.

- Insurance policies are either too restrictive or expensive. "Cadillac" policies, purchased at high costs, cover most expenses, including dental and vision insurance. While such coverage is desirable, most U.S. citizens cannot afford it.

- The high cost of health care exacerbates the cost of insurance.

- The economic recession has left millions without health insurance.

- When people lose jobs, they usually lose health care insurance.

- Half of all home foreclosures are related to health care costs.[18]

- Profit-driven health insurance overshadows moral considerations. Annual CEO compensation for 2011 ranged from $7.3 million (Humana) to $19 million (Cigna): http://bit.ly/insurance-ceos ("Insurance Carriers").

- The many profit players in health care and malpractice insurance for providers make health care costly.

- Bankruptcies continue to increase. An estimated 60 percent of bankruptcies are due to medical bills (NBC newscast, July 21, 2009, reported

---

[18]Christopher T. Robertson, Richard Egelhof, and Michael Hoke, "Get Sick, Get Out: The Medical Causes of Home Mortgage Foreclosures," *Health Matrix: Journal of Law–Medicine* 18, no. 65 (2008), http://ssrn.com/abstract=1416947. Abstract: from a study done in four states, nearly half of all respondents (49%) indicated that their home foreclosures were due in part to costly medical problems of various types. This datum also appears in the U.S. Affordable Care Act.

it at two-thirds). In 2009 75 percent of those declaring bankruptcy did so as a result of medical bills or lack of health insurance.[19]

EXTENDING HEALTH CARE ACCESS

Most developed countries provide health care for everyone regardless of their ability to pay (true even for Rwanda).[20] In the United States those enrolled in Social Security and who are sixty-six and over may receive Medicare coverage (Plans A and B), a form of universal health care for a select portion of the population. This provision began July 30, 1965, with an amendment signed by President Johnson.[21] The United States is the only wealthy, industrialized nation that does not provide universal health care.

In light of Bazzana's research on the differences in the early Roman Empire between physician's fees in the West and the East of the empire (see chap. 3), the same pattern continues today, only the West and East each extend 6,000 miles further beyond the Roman Empire's western and eastern boundaries. In the empire's West physicians received relatively good incomes from a health tax (*iatrikon*) *and* fees for service; in the East the medical personnel's income was much lower, but physicians were held in high honor with prestige in the community. T. R. Reid's comparison of the health care systems of the United States and Japan demonstrates the same West-East differential. Japan has a mix of private and public health care, but not a citizen choice between the two. All citizens participate in both. In Japan people visit their doctors more often than anywhere else in the world (fourteen times annually on average). They might take a small gift, as a symbol of honor for their physician. The salaries of medical personnel are much lower than in the United States, but doctors are highly esteemed. If Reid had his shoulder

---

[19]Based on a CNN "Money and Main Street" newscast, June 5, 2009. Author Steffie Woolhandler, of the Harvard Medical School, writes in the *American Journal of Medicine* "that 62.1 percent of the bankruptcies were medically related because the individuals either had more than $5,000 (or 10 percent of their pretax income) in medical bills, mortgaged their home to pay for medical bills, or lost significant income due to an illness. On average, medically bankrupt families had $17,943 in out-of-pocket expenses, including $26,971 for those who lacked insurance and $17,749 who had insurance at some point."

[20]For the national system of health care in Rwanda, see Fareed Zakaria, "Africa's New Path: Paul Kagame Charts a Way Forward," *Newsweek*, July 17, 2009, p. 26.

[21]The costs of Medicare and Medicaid now play into current debates over the federal budget and deficit. Medicare programs began in Australia in 1970 and in Canada 1966-1984.

replacement done in Japan, it would have cost him one-fourth as much as in the United States.[22] His copay would have been $650. His clinic call cost $94 with insurance covering all but $19 (his copay).[23] Japan's health care outcomes are some of the highest in the world. "Japan leads the world in life expectancy (85.5 years for women, 78.7 for men) and in the more relevant statistic, healthy life expectancy at age sixty."[24]

Like the United States, Japan is capitalist, but the medical percent of their GDP is less than half that of the United States (8%).[25] Japan's 3,500 health insurance companies are linked to either employer companies or municipalities. These plans fall into three different categories: large companies pay 55 percent of the insurance cost; smaller companies split the cost half and half for employers and employees. All others have Citizens Health Insurance where the local government and the patient split the cost.[26] The government mandate of health insurance for all is not controversial. It's considered every person's responsibility.[27] The public aspect of Japan's health care system is that the government sets the fees for all services and procedures. Insurance companies reimburse medical personnel promptly—no hassle!

Perhaps the United States can learn from Japan how to make health care more efficient and friendly. If combined with France's *cart vitale*—"a green plastic card with a small gold memory chip" that retains the patient's medical records[28]—eliminating space-and-time-consuming files and filing, the *ideal* system could be had! The United States could simplify its private health care system and provide quality (value) care with efficiency.[29] The health care systems of Australia, Germany (the Bismarck model) or

---

[22]T. R. Reid, *The Healing of America: A Global Quest for Better, Cheaper, and Fairer Health Care* (New York: Penguin, 2009), p. 83.

[23]Ibid., p. 86.

[24]Ibid., pp. 84-85.

[25]Ibid., p. 85.

[26]Ibid., pp. 86-87.

[27]Ibid., p. 87.

[28]Ibid., p. 49.

[29]My own recent experiences testify to this waste of time: twenty minutes checking my meds when admitted to E.R., and then several hours later the same procedure occurs upon admittance to the hospital, followed by the same tabulation of meds again when visiting my new primary care doctor. On each visit the same process is repeated, even though I present a typed page listing my meds and current dosage each time. Finding a patient's records in the voluminous office files occupies a significant portion of a person's time.

Switzerland (next costly to the United States), however, may be more conducive to the U.S. economy and its health care reform.[30]

The advantages of a single-payer system are reducing layers of expense and profit in the system, making health care affordable for all, and achieving greater efficiency in every medical-related office. The disadvantages are whether a huge government bureaucracy can be efficient and pay claims in a timely manner, whether the amount paid adequately covers costs and provides acceptable salaries for health care professionals, and whether we have enough primary care doctors to serve the millions now uninsured. The pros and cons of these issues need to be fairly debated.

The massive contribution of Michael Porter and Elizabeth Omsted Teisberg explains the rationale for and charts the path toward the goal of value-based and quality-care competition.[31] Of the many aspects of systemic change Porter and Teisberg call for, I mention four of their nine changes under one section, "Restructure the Health Plan-Provider Relationship":

• *Shift the nature of information sharing with providers.* Ways must be developed so that listening is two-way: doctors listen to what patients have to say about their condition and their perception of it as well as vice versa. Health plans must be structured to take this into account. This will enhance preventive care. More attention to preventing illness is perhaps the most important factor facing health care. But it is not easy to shift medical service from "curing" to "preventing."[32]

• *Reward provider excellence and value-enhancing innovation.* Beginning in 2011 Medicare and Anthem have moved in the direction of rewarding value performance by allowing higher compensation for those providers that score high on forty-eight standards of measurement, compared to peers in the system.[33]

---

[30]Universal health coverage began in the U.K. in 1948.

[31]Michael Porter and Elizabeth Omsted Teisberg, *Redefining Health Care: Creating Value-Based Competition on Results* (Boston: Harvard Business School Press, 2006), pp. 97-148. See the list of "imperatives for providers" in figure 5-1, p. 157.

[32]In an insightful contribution, Schumpeter has identified this issue as crucial and calls for creative incentives to assist people toward prevention, citing a South African company that gives air miles for exercising and buying healthy foods (Schumpeter, "Getting on the Treadmill," *The Economist*, October 8, 2011, p. 80).

[33]Information from Jenn Burkett, director of Total Value Management at Elkhart General Hospital.

- *Move to single bills for episodes and cycles of care, and single prices.* This contrasts with separate billing for each item and provider (doctor, hospital, pills, equipment used, etc.). This change requires substantial overhaul of the present system since billing comes from separate financial entities. However, the September 23, 2011, one-year anniversary report on the achievements of the Affordable Care Act refers to this as "bundled payments" and says initiatives that have put this into practice have shown that this change "can improve health, improve the quality of care, and lower costs."[34] Though gains in all three areas are salutary in the Geisinger Health System, numerous hurdles must be overcome to enact this approach more broadly.[35]

- Simplify, standardize, and eliminate paperwork and transactions. Reduce paperwork for all involved.[36]

Many features of the health care system that Porter and Teisberg mention have already become operational in several medical centers: Mayo Clinic, the Cleveland Clinic and the Geisinger Health system in northeast Pennsylvania. The gains in quality and cost reduction in the Geisinger model is salutary: "750 physicians . . . serve 2.6 million patients across 43 counties."[37] While health care reform has become a divisive issue in the U.S. political climate, most agree that we need to find ways to reduce rising costs.[38]

In his *Memoirs* Joseph Martin, retired dean of Harvard Medical School and earlier chancellor of the University of California–San Francisco School of Medicine, identifies three areas of needed change to progress toward a sustainable health care system. First, reduce health

---

[34]In the section on "Investing in Innovation, Improving Care and Saving Money" in the "Reducing Costs, Protecting Consumers: Affordable Care Act on the One Year Anniversary of the Patient's Bill of Rights," *HealthCare.gov*, September 23, 2011, www.healthcare.gov/law/resources/reports/patients-bill-of-rights09232011a.pdf.

[35]Robert E. Mechanic, "Opportunities and Challenges for Episode-Based Payment," *The New England Journal of Medicine* 365 (2011): 777-79.

[36]Porter and Teisberg, *Redefining Health Care*, pp. 258-68.

[37]Patricia Barry, "The New Face of Health Care: A new system rewards doctors and hospitals for taking better care of patients at lower costs." AARP Bulletin, April 1, 2009. Available at www.aarp.org/health/doctors-hospitals/info-04-2009/the_new_face_of_health_care.html

[38]Some researchers believe that health care costs could be reduced by a stunning 30 percent—or about $700 billion a year—without harming quality if we moved as a nation toward the proven and successful practices adopted by health care providers and hospitals in the lower medical costs areas.

care costs by having all insurance companies adopt a standardized form for filing claims, thereby cutting administrative costs. Second, provide incentives for more primary care doctors, reducing the ratio between lower cost care and higher cost care with so many different specialties. Third, move from fee-for-service to salaried doctors; costs are less and quality outcomes are better.[39]

INITIAL NATIONAL HEALTH CARE REFORMS

The Patient Protection and Affordable Care Act (Title I) identifies specific areas to promote wellness and prevention of disease: "(1) Smoking cessation; (2) Weight management; (3) Stress management; (4) Physical fitness; (5) Nutrition; (6) Heart disease prevention; (7) Healthy lifestyle support; and (8) Diabetes prevention."[40] The two integrated health care bills, with parts taking effect September 23, 2010, address the three components at the core of the U.S. health care crisis: *cost*, *quality* and *access*. Unfortunately, this document does not include *violence prevention*, which is identified by the World Health Organization as a key factor in health care costs. Violence of any kind, especially wars, increases national health care budgets exponentially![41]

A one-year anniversary release identifies numerous benefits achieved by the Patient Protection and Affordable Care Act in the first year:

- The Patient's Bill of Rights makes it illegal for insurance industries to deny coverage to children with preexisting conditions. Lifetime dollar limits on coverage is also illegal.

---

[39] Joseph B. Martin, *From Alfalfa to Ivy: Memoirs of a Harvard Medical School Dean* (Edmonton, Alberta, Can.: University of Alberta Press, 2011), pp. 361-68. Martin's second point is reinforced by an article that points out that in 1960 the U.S. had 18 specialty boards with a handful of subspecialties. In 2011 there are 158 specialties and subspecialties (compared to Canada, 67; France, 52; England, 97), with a shortage in primary care physicians. See Allan S. Detsky, M.D., Ph.D., Stephen R. Ganthier, B.Sc., Victor R. Fuchs, Ph.D., "Specialization in Medicine: How Much Is Appropriate?" in *The Journal of the American Medical Association*, February 1, 2012, p. 463.

[40] "Patient Protection and Affordable Care Act: Title I. Quality, Affordable Health Care for All Americans," May 1, 2010, p. 39, www.healthcare.gov/law/full/.

[41] Here I lump together the health care costs of all violence: domestic, various daily types headlining local newspapers, and the care of wounded war veterans that affect health care budgets. For the cost of veterans' health care alone, one of the larger components of the U.S. budget, see "Veteran's Health Care Costs Are a Big Part of Federal Budget," *Kaiser Health News*, July 28, 2011, www.kaiserhealthnews.org/daily-reports/2011/july/28/vets-health-care-costs.aspx.

- The Affordable Care Act has created the "Pre-existing Condition Insurance Plan" (PCIP) to make health insurance available to those previously denied because of preexisting conditions. Over 30,000 people have already benefited from this provision.

- One million young adults received health insurance through coverage under their parent's private health insurance.

- Seniors who hit the donut hole on drugs received a 50 percent discount on brand name drugs. Nearly 1.3 million have benefited during this first year of implementation.

- Small businesses with fewer than twenty-five full-time workers qualified for a tax credit of up to 35 percent, which in 2014 will increase to 50 percent.

- Health insurance companies are required to spend 80 to 85 percent for large group markets—of premium dollars on health care, not overhead, advertising, and bonuses. This expense for the insurance industry is the Medical Loss Ratio (MLR)! Over 165 million have received better value for their insurance dollars since this ruling took effect on September 23, 2010.

- Nearly 19 million seniors have received free preventive services and 1.3 million, a free annual wellness visit.[42]

No longer do we need to carry the guilt of depriving health care to those who need it most, those with preexisting conditions. Fundamental problems continue to strain the economics of providing health care, however. The cost of health care continues to rise. Since President Obama's proposed "public option" was defeated, the inclusion of many more people in the insurance pool in the next years assures rising market profit of the health insurance companies, even though the reform act assumes reduced

---

[42]"Patient Protection and Affordable Care Act: Title I. Quality, Affordable Health Care for All Americans," May 1, 2010, p. 39, www.healthcare.gov/law/full/. CBS News, "Los Angeles lines up for free medical care" (October 24, 2011), showed lines of people who came overnight to L.A.'s Memorial Arena waiting for this free annual preventative care checkup, including dental and vision. Many have no health insurance and for the first time in years now received dental and vision care. Eighty doctors and many other medical personnel helped with this event, sponsored by the nonprofit Care Now. Over 3700 people received this service on October 24, in a city with two million uninsured residents. www.cbsnews.com/video/watch/?id=7385837n.

costs through large-scale efficiencies.[43] One political conservative, R. R. Reno, assesses the reform law and finds much good in it, too readily dismissed by its opponents. From his religious perspective he regards paying for abortions as bad.[44] Then he says,

> But what about the rest of the bill? The Democrats did not so much change the American health-care system as they rather pumped up everything in an attempt to realize the imperative of universal access. Some Christians, including politically conservative Christians warmly welcome this.[45]

He foresees the outcome as a boost to the health care system financially and morally. Health insurance companies will have more clients which should enable lower premiums for all. The fear of federally bloated costs need not be the outcome. The proposal enhances economic growth.

I regard universal coverage for basic health care a biblical moral priority. But the complexity of the U.S. system makes it hard to achieve. The Patient Protection and Affordable Care Act projects a virtual achievement of that goal by 2021. I hope it works. Everyone, rich and poor alike, deserves equal health care access, regardless of race, creed, class, marital status, gender identity or other differences that mark our society, unless for conscience reasons they opt out of the system, including Social Security and Medicare, as the Amish do. The Amish model attracts some but represents a small fraction of the U.S. population. They pay for their health care by raising money for expenses in their local and neighboring districts, and then appealing to Amish districts in other states when costs are too high for districts in one state to bear.

OTHER FACTORS AND CONSIDERATIONS

In a report of health care expense for the year 2003, the United States spends almost twice as much per capita for health care as do any of these countries: Canada, the United Kingdom, Japan and Germany. The average life expectancy age is higher for both women and men in these coun-

---

[43]Walmart's need to trim insurance coverage for its employees and raise the premiums (see n. 14 earlier) casts doubt that large-scale efficiency results in lower insurance premiums. Perhaps Walmart's insured employee-pool, however, has higher than the national average of medical expenses, producing a greater medical loss on its insurance balance sheet.

[44]R. R. Reno, "Reforming the Health-Care Reform," *First Things*, June–July 2010, pp. 61-63.

[45]Ibid., p. 61.

tries than it is in the United States. "A 2004 study by HealthGrades estimated that 195,000 die each year in U.S. hospitals because of preventable
treatment errors."[46] Will the implementation of the Affordable Care Act
change these facts and enable the United States to gain standing above its
rating in 2000 as 37th in health care performance among the nations of
the world?

Morally, biblically and theologically we must do better in light of our
medical and technological expertise. Can the costs of health care be reduced without a fundamental rethinking of the relation between health
care and the market-driven system the United States presently has? Will
larger scale insurance operations result in cost reductions, as projected?
The Institute of Medicine (IOM), which has been charged with the Congressional mandate to the Department of Health and Human Services
(DHHS) to develop a profile of "'essential health benefits' (EHBs) equiv-
alent to that of a 'typical employer plan,' does not forecast premium reductions under the Affordable Care Act, but premium increases in the 'Individual Market.'"[47]

T. R. Reid's book title *The Healing of America* signals the deeper nature
of the problem.[48] Our way of thinking about health care, which is so much
the victim of economic greed and political rancor, identifies just how
steeped we are in an entitlement and profit-making approach to health
care. This problem raises the need for conversion in desire and expectations, sharing of resources and loving care for the sick that has characterized the church's mission through the ages. Health care as mission must
take priority over drive for profit margins.

We must continue the quest to improve health and health care in the
United States. While we applaud impressive advances in medical technology
and treatment, which have done much to cure disease and ease suffering, we

---

[46]Porter and Teisberg, *Redefining Health Care*, p. 22. Based on a 2003 study that Porter and
Teisberg present in graph form on the huge gap between "recommended appropriate care and
delivered care by specific condition" (ibid., p. 23). See also Barbara Starfield, "America's
Health Care System Is the Third Leading Cause of Death," summarized by Kah Ying Choo,
Journal of the American Medical Association 284, no. 4 (2000): 483-85.

[47]John K. Iglehart, "Defining Essential Health Benefits—The View from the IOM Committee," *The New England Journal of Medicine* 365 (2011): 1461-63. See also Paul B. Ginsburg,
"Reforming Provider Payment—The Price Side of the Equation," *The New England Journal of
Medicine* 365 (2011): 1268-70. Medicare and Medicaid pay less to hospitals for services than
private insurers do.

[48]T. R. Reid's study of health care systems worldwide is an engaging and sobering read.

must own the fact that the United States health care has been unjustly distributed, broken and unsustainable. While the health care crisis is indeed an economic and political issue, it is also a moral, ethical and ultimately spiritual issue.[49] And this we must own, address and seek to correct.

In an extensive analysis of health care ethics, combining philosophical and evangelical moral perspectives, James Thobaben contends that U.S. health care has moved from "a covenantal relation" between practitioner and patient to a "social contract," in which both the practitioner and patient have expected roles and "rights."[50] Modern philosophical values of individualism and autonomy forced health care to shift to the social-contract model. While his book is heavy-going at points, especially in its philosophical analysis, it provides many useful insights on what the rights of both providers and patients are within the social-contract model. His analysis of how "sickness" is understood from an ethical perspective in social contract is enlightening, especially when he examines HIV/AIDS: how it fits the sickness model in medical treatment and social understanding and how it does not.[51]

Medical ethics is a vast topic with many angles of contribution.[52] Though this book does not take up this topic in depth, others do. One of the best introductions to the field is *Theological Voices in Medical Ethics*, edited by Allen Verhey and Stephen Lammers.[53] In it David Smith examines Paul Ramsey's thoughtful analysis of the topic under the title "A

---

[49]The work of Dr. Jim Withers in Pittsburgh providing health care to the homeless (living under the bridge of the I-376 overpass) since 1992 is a shining testimony. Withers says, "The essence of healthcare is going to where people are. Either physically or even more importantly spiritually, emotionally." Under Operation Safety Net, seven hundred homeless people have been housed in empty apartments as a result of his initiatives, courage, and compassion (CBS News, October 21, 2011), www.cbs.com/sitesearch/results/?q=Jim+Withers%2C+Oct+21%2C+2011. Thank God for Dr. Withers and his kind!

[50]James R. Thobaben, *Health-Care Ethics: A Comprehensive Guide* (Downers Grove, Ill.: IVP Academic, 2009), pp. 135-79. His method is instructive. Part one of each chapter focuses on selected Scriptures and their significance for the topic under discussion. Part two examines the topic from a Christian (evangelical) perspective. Part three takes up the same aspect of bioethics from the perspective of the "Christian and the world." In this latter part he connects the social-contract model to his ethical proposals.

[51]Ibid., pp. 176-78.

[52]For an exhaustive treatment, with many contributors, see *On Moral Medicine: Theological Perspectives in Medical Ethics*, ed. M. Theresa Lysaught and Joseph J. Kotva Jr. with Stephen Lammers and Allen Verhey (Grand Rapids: Eerdmans, 2012).

[53]Allen Verhey and Stephen Lammers, ed., *Theological Voices in Medical Ethics* (Grand Rapids: Eerdmans, 1993).

Covenant-Centered Ethic for Medicine."[54] This is intriguing in light of Thobaben's proposal that current medical ethics beyond the church must proceed in its analysis with the social-contract model, for the covenant model no longer holds sway. Verhey considers James Gustafson's contribution at length under the title "Can Medical Ethics Be Christian?"[55] Lammers follows up with an analysis of Stanley Hauerwas's contribution under the title "Theology, Medical Ethics, and the Church."[56] A later chapter by Marc Gellman, "Bringing the Ancient Word to the Modern World" is most instructive in that it discusses both philosophical perspectives and current ethical issues such as abortion.[57]

Three major challenges confront the U.S. health care system as it wends its way into the future. First, we must seek to move from "defensive medicine" to "good medicine"—that which produces the best outcomes for patient health (see chap. 11 for more on defensive medicine). Second, since health care has become a commodity, with manufacturers selling "products" and patients becoming "consumers," we must convert our thinking about what health care is and why it exists. Let's not forget history (chap. 8) and what it teaches us about the church's primary role in health care.

Third, we must overcome the disconnect that exists in today's health care system. Patients often don't know what prescribed tests cost, and doctors who prescribe them don't know either. The same applies to prescribed drugs, though a question about this by the patient usually elicits an answer, sometimes after research. Patients and doctors need to think how their decisions affect the entire system's cost, and not only whether it is covered by insurance. Only then can we break the spiraling cycle of runaway costs.

Answers to the issues posed by medicine and medical practice in our modern world are not easy. We can nevertheless recover in part the covenantal contract by joining the prayers of the church to the work of health care providers.

---

[54]David Smith, "A Covenant-Centered Ethic for Medicine," in *Theological Voices in Medical Ethics*, pp. 7-29.

[55]Allen Verhey, "Can Medical Ethics Be Christian?" in *Theological Voices in Medical Ethics*, pp. 30-56.

[56]Stephen Lammers, "Theology, Medical Ethics, and the Church," in *Theological Voices in Medical Ethics*, pp. 57-77.

[57]Marc Gellman, "Bringing the Ancient Word to the Modern World," in *Theological Voices in Medical Ethics*, pp. 178-208.

MEDITATION, FOR SPIRITUAL REFLECTION AND PRAYER

Let us pray for those who do not have health care.

Let us pray for health care providers.

Let us pray for all in leadership positions. . . .

[May they] point the way to solutions

that assure . . . the care . . . people need.

Let us pray for the sick and injured.

Let us pray for ourselves . . .

for health, for caring hands to reach out, for loving

hearts to share another's pain, for the will to solve big problems.

We pray these things with gratitude for the life you have given us,

     for your care that enfolds us and for your love made known on the
     cross. Amen.[58]

---

[58]Worship resources, July 19, 2009, from Mennonite Central Committee, Washington, D.C., Office. This prayer resembles some parts of Walter Rauschenbusch's prayer written over a hundred years ago for medical personnel and friends who care for us when we are afflicted with sickness. Allen Verhey begins part two of *Remembering Jesus* with this lengthy prayer (pp. 79-80). Part two is titled "Remembering Jesus in the Strange World of Sickness: A Continuing Tradition of Care for the Suffering." (Allen Verhey, *Remembering Jesus: Christian Community, Scripture, and the Moral Life* [Grand Rapids: Eerdmans, 2002], pp. 77-154.)

11

❖

From High Tech and Triage to Shalom and Service

Because health is a gift from God and our bodies are temples of the Holy Spirit, we seek to be better stewards of our health. . . . [W]e commit ourselves to work toward adequate access to health care for all our brothers and sisters. . . . [W]e will work as stewards of the gospel to provide better health care access for our neighbors. . . . [W]e will be advocates on behalf of public health matters and access to health care for everyone.

Health Care Access Statement of Mennonite Church USA

People of Christian faith might readily make these commitments:

1. affirm biblical beliefs about life and death, including hope in the resurrection

2. strive to make the congregation a healing community

3. educate ourselves on issues of healing, wellness, advance medical directives, health care ethics and health care alternatives

4. recognize and affirm the ministry and accountability of health care institutions, health care professionals and other care givers

5. recover commitment to community through a graduated cost-scale for health care

6. become advocates for a health care system that includes fairness, accountability and accessibility

7. encourage our church health-related organizations to help members understand and guide response to health care needs

High Tech and Triage

These two important heath care practices function as foils for addressing ethical issues in health care. Health care providers know on a daily basis the meaning of high tech and triage. They know the valuable contribution of high-tech interventions and they know the importance of triage in sorting out which situations take priority. My own E.R. visits with heart illness have demonstrated its importance and excellence.

In this chapter, however, I use *triage* in a different specific sense, that is, giving priority to those who *are able to pay* for their health care and denying health care to the uninsured or underinsured. Those who cannot pay are either referred elsewhere or not treated at all. The people who need health care most may thus not have access to it. That is our present system's form of rationing, subservient to "market economics." Complaints about rationing health care if and as the Affordable Care Act is implemented overlook the fact that rationing is and has been operative in U.S. health care practices over the past years, often in cruel and unfair forms, like when an insurance company drops one of its insured when major medical expenses mount or are forecast. Further, denying to the uninsured health care they cannot afford is systemic rationing.

High tech now plays a dominant role in U.S. health care. High tech, with its promising potential, also has a downside. To illustrate how high tech can contribute to or impede good health, I cite a story from an informal discussion in the seminary lounge where I taught for twenty-six years. Speaking about his wife's pregnancy and the medical counsel she was receiving about the mother's role in the delivery process, a male student developed negative feelings about high tech. He said that with all our high-tech efforts to assist in deliveries, the infant mortality rate in the United States has not come down significantly. It is still the highest among the developed nations of the world. Why go to the expense of high-tech equipment for delivery (what procedure was used is not clear), when the same result is achieved with eight minutes of more work? High tech increases expense, but may not improve the overall health care experience of the birthing mother. Other factors such as the husband's presence, caring expertise on the part of doctors and nurses, and overall positive psychological and spiritual support for the birthing mother are more important to a wholesome experience.

Ordinary people are often frustrated with not knowing how to respond to high-tech procedures and interventions. Dr. Glen Miller's book provides helpful guidance in navigating the system.[1] Many people, however, are grateful that a particular intervention either saved their lives or contributed to their quality of life. A pacemaker-defibrillator implanted in 2005 six years after my heart attack and again in 2010 is a case in point. High tech often produces desirable results, but it must be assessed within a larger analysis of health care systems. The temptation to order all tests possibly relevant—sometimes by different doctors on the case and overlapping in function—is hard to resist when and if medical salaries or bonuses are enhanced on that basis. High tech is a Catch-22, since lives are saved through its use by skilled medical expertise.

But do the uninsured and underinsured receive the same benefits and quality of care as those with insurance? Some doctors refuse Medicare/Medicaid patients, since capped reimbursement negatively affects the profit line. Too often the uninsured are racially skewed: one in four Hispanics, one in five African Americans but only one in ten Anglos or other. Most are from the lower socioeconomic class. In light of such statistics it is clear that triage is pervasively at work in health care access. Can our health care system be more inclusive, advancing its benefits for all people when they need it?

SHALOM AND COMMUNITY

Dr. Willard Krabill spoke of "the devil's triangle," the interrelationship of three factors: access, quality and cost (see chap. 6). The health care debate revolves around these issues. Some argue that while we may have two of these at any given time, we cannot have all three together. Krabill challenges that conclusion and argues for a concept of quality that makes access and cost copartners with quality. In chapter six I proposed another triangle, "God's shalom triangle," to complement our health care system. The values, indeed Christian virtues, in this triangle are community, mutual sharing and justice/compassion. In this triangle each element is a necessary component of the other. Each supports and enhances the other.

The biblical view of health is holistic, fostering shalom. *Shalom* repu-

---

[1]Glen E. Miller, *Empowering the Patient: How to Reduce the Cost of Health Care and Improve Its Quality* (Indianapolis: Dog Ear, 2009).

diates any soul-body distinction and embraces the material, social, psychological, physical and spiritual dimensions of life. Most scholarly work on shalom has overlooked the importance of *health* as part of shalom.[2] *Shalom* as "well-being" is explicit in shalom's cognate, *shalem* (occurring thirty-three times in the Old Testament), which denotes holistic health, "wellness." *Shalem* connotes the sense of "single eye" (i.e., no duplicity). Clarity in values, without conflicting loyalties, and basic honesty are important ingredients of *shalem* health. Distortion of truth, confusion of thought and values, or saying one thing and doing another threaten and ultimately destroy *shalem* health in persons and community. When these destructive behaviors characterize systems and societal structures their destructive power is even greater, even though subtle and less readily perceived. Our pace of life works against the centering of spirit and emotion that *shalem* requires. Hence we need sabbath time for rest and renewal.[3]

Chapter six includes extended discussion on the meaning of *shalom*.[4] One crucial supportive component of shalom is *community*. The role of community and its relation to health occurred in almost every chapter: in thesis 1 of chapter 1; the "focal images" at the end of chapter two; the "God as Healer" section in chapter three; the third paradox in chapter four; the whole of chapter five; its relation to God's shalom triangle in chapter six; and the frontispiece on mutual aid in chapter seven. In the third paradox (in chap. 4) *community* is essential for countering human alienation, emptiness, loneliness and despair. God's gift of community koinonia) in the fellowship of the Holy Spirit, with common faith, hope and love, enables peace and purpose to life. The William Walsh and John Langan quotation introducing chapter seven rightly identifies community as "the one distinctive gift of [early] Christianity." This bonding of Jesus' followers to one another enabled them to survive persecution,

---

[2]Introducing the extensive bibliography on *shalom* and *eirēnē* in *The Meaning of Peace*, I noted that if biblical scholarship had included health/healing in shalom, the present bibliography would be incomplete ("Introduction to the Bibliography," *The Meaning of Peace*, ed. Perry Yoder and Willard Swartley, rev. ed. [Elkhart, Ind.: Institute of Mennonite Studies, 2001], p. 260).

[3]Tilden Edwards, who heads up the Shalem Institute in Washington, D.C., develops this point in his excellent book *Sabbath Time: Understanding and Practice for Contemporary Christians* (New York: Seabury Press, 1982).

[4]In Hebrew Scripture *shalom* embraces salvation, justice and peace. See Perry B. Yoder, *Shalom: The Bible's Word for Salvation, Justice, and Peace* (Nappanee, Ind.: Evangel, 1997), pp. 3-52.

indeed not only to survive but to grow and thrive.

Commitment to community naturally leads to practice of mutual aid, so that economic and health care needs are met with caring love for one another. As appendix two demonstrates, a Christian community of churches working together can make health care available to the uninsured. Community identity provides also an inner peace and stability when life is chaotic, when poverty, oppression and violence befall us. In his summary report of a twelve-year study by an interdisciplinary team of scholars, Ulrich Luz describes the team's conclusion regarding peace in relation to experiences of violence, poverty and oppression. One of the unexpected conclusions of the study is that while the biblical teaching opposes oppression, poverty and violence, it also values another reality:

> It is no accident that in all of the essays [from this twelve-year study] the so-called "inner dimension" played a notable role. All the participants found it necessary to add a fourth dimension to the three dimensions of peace identified at the outset of this study ([minimization of] poverty, violence, and oppression). [This fourth dimension] they describe variously as "minimization of fear," of "sin," with "comfort," or "gaining of identity." In virtually all the studies it became clear that this inner dimension need not stand as a contrast to the outer dimensions of peace. Forgiveness of debt, the lifting of fear, experiencing comfort, and gaining of identity, do not replace active expressions of peacemaking, but rather enable them. It became evident that the inner and the outer are modern points of contrast whereas in biblical anthropology they are integrated.[5]

This inner dimension of peace is much related to community. Early Christian believers knew peace—some sense of shalom—even when the larger world they lived in was racked with injustice, war and violence. When facing sickness and plagues, an inner peace and wholeness gave comfort and strength (see chap. 7). This strikes a somber but joyful note: we need not wait until the United States solves its health care crisis or the world its injustices until we can experience, to some extent at least, God's shalom and wholeness, through the strength and caring love of Christian community.

---

[5]Ulrich Luz, "The Significance of the Biblical Witness for Church Peace Action," in *The Meaning of Peace*, ed. Perry B. Yoder, and Willard M. Swartley, 2nd ed. (Elkhart, Ind.: Institute of Mennonite Studies, 2001), pp. 238-39.

For treatment of *mutual aid*, the second pole in God's shalom triangle, see chapter seven.

THE JUSTICE PERSPECTIVE

The justice tradition is strong in biblical thought. (See biblical theme 2 and the comments on justice in relation to God's shalom triangle in chap. 6.) The semantic field of justice is steadfast love, faithfulness, righteousness and peace. Righteousness and justice often occur in parallel lines or are "twined" in the Psalms and the Prophets.

> Steadfast love and faithfulness will meet;
>   righteousness and peace will kiss each other. (Ps 85:10)

> Righteousness and justice are the foundation of your throne;
>   steadfast love and faithfulness go before you. (Ps 89:14)

Each of these divine attributes complements the others. These divine virtues are understood as accessible to and attainable by.Israel through faithful covenant with God.

Willard Krabill contends that health care is one of the church's foremost justice concerns. From a Christian theological-ethical perspective our response to the health care crisis must be motivated by concern for justice as part of peacemaking. Jesus did not restrict the scope of his healing to the ritually clean, or to Jews only (chap. 3). His healing ministry tilted toward inclusion of those classified as "sinners" in and outside of Israel. The biblical, theological and ethical tradition speaks strongly against injustice: the community of faith cares for the resident alien, orphans, widows and the poor. Justice and compassion respond to those in need of basic health care.

To illustrate an injustice that stifles shalom, I refer to a mildly charismatic Christian surgeon living outside the United States but in an affiliated country making $800,000 annually in 1992. He built a luxurious house for his family, even though he lives among poor people. He benefits from the Medicaid system and charges additional fees when he can. He is skilled and well liked. This poses an ethical problem. Christian practitioners need to exemplify a different model. Might dedicated Christian practitioners set limits to their income and pass that benefit on to the needy?

In 1993 the Associated Press reported on an interview with doctors about their salaries. The average medical doctor's salary at that time was

$172,000. Some earned up to $750,000-$1,000,000 annually. One surgeon, with income in that range in 1993 at a medical conference where I spoke, told me he works hard and deserves it. Perhaps a sustainable resolution of the health care crisis requires salary caps for medical practitioners and health insurance employees, especially for CEOs and CFOs whose salaries far surpass that of medical providers and their employees generally.[6]

Setting salary limits, however, may jeopardize the quality and motivation of service. Salary increases can function as positive incentives. Hence, a "profit, efficiency, cost reduction" triangle can benefit both patients and the health care system. In this triangle each component enables the next component of the triangle, in that order. The motivation of profit or increased salary leads to greater efficiency, which in turn saves total costs in the health care system, when demand exceeds personnel resources.

The theological basis for profit-motivation appeals to thesis 1 of chapter one: Our creation in the divine image means we are to exercise dominion over all creation and at the same time value community. The dominion stewardship of creation is the cultural mandate involving work, creative invention, managing, preserving and tending (Gen 2:15). Community and dominion (tending creation) are essential components of health.

This view is tenable and has merit, depending largely on the conscientiousness of the provider. Even so, limits to income may be necessary for the sake of making the health care system sustainable and enhancing the other component in the creation mandate: community. While doctors' salaries have remained relatively flat compared to other rising living costs in the last twenty years (e.g., gasoline and health insurance premiums), a wide range of incomes exists. Physicians' salaries may vary from as low as $80,000 (or lower) annually for primary care providers (PCPs) in underserved areas to as high as $1,000,000 (and higher) for specialists in urban areas where costs of living are high. The cost of malpractice insurance can vary also from $10,000 (or lower) to nearly $200,000 (for ObGyn) in Florida, for example.

Some limits, preferably self-imposed, are essential because human greed readily takes over, evident in the financial scandals exposed in the

---

[6]Recall how the federal government capped salaries of bank CEOs when receiving TARP money.

economic collapse of 2007-2009.[7] When internal moral restraints cease to function, external controls are needed. Some evidence indicates that when doctors are salaried the overall performance is rated higher for quality care (even though they may do fewer tests, which use expensive technology).[8] The Affordable Care Act mandates that compensation for services be linked to quality care.[9] Cost control will be effective only when it is systemwide, not just tweaking Medicare eligibility age, for example.[10]

The Japanese health care system might instruct us. Based on a 2007 source, the Japanese use high tech readily, at that time doing three times as many MRIs as in the United States (MRI prescription, however, has

---

[7]For an insightful critique of greed and its economic consequences for health care, see the article by Peter M. Carney, M.D., neurosurgeon and Fellow of the American Association of Neurological Surgeons, "Is Greed Good???" paper presented at the Medical Ethics Conference at the University of Notre Dame, Notre Dame, Ind., March 2-4, 2012. Carney first notes that some medical practitioners view greed as good since it promotes innovation and medical inventions for human good. He cites Cardinal Tariscio Bertone who in July 2009 stated that "the free market had been replaced by the 'greed market,' which then caused the 2007-08 world wide financial crisis." Carney does not define greed, but notes that theologians through the centuries, e.g., Thomas Aquinas, regarded greed as a cardinal sin. While definition is difficult in a capitalist economy, Scripture (Col 3:5; Eph 5:5) names greed idolatry. I suggest then greed is the desire and passion to accumulate wealth and material possessions as *the chief focus* of one's life. However, wealth may be a blessing of the Lord, as Psalm 112:3 attests. Such people fear the Lord, are gracious and merciful, generously lend, conduct their affairs with justice, distribute freely, and give to the poor (vv. 1, 4-5, 9).

Carney refers to an article by Dr. Robert Brook in *The Journal of the American Medical Association* (August 2011) titled "The Role of Physicians in Controlling Medical Care Costs and Reducing Waste." Carney says Brook contends that "because cost of medical care is increasing faster than the gross domestic product (GDP) and the federal deficit is increasing, many economists believe that the federal *'deficit cannot be reduced unless medical spending can be controlled.'* Dr. Brook describes three *'scenarios'* for physicians in controlling health care costs. First, do nothing. Costs continue to rise *'unabated'* and sooner or later solutions will be applied that are not what *'physicians, or their patients, want.'* In the second *'scenario,'* health care is *'rationed.'* At the mere mention of the R word *'all rational discussion ceases'* so that this solution becomes one that *'most individuals would like to avoid.'* In the third *'scenario'* physicians take *'the lead in identifying and eliminating waste in US health care.'"* Carney's conclusion is that medical schools and organizations such as Notre Dame's Center for Ethics and Culture must encourage physicians to pursue the "Art of Medicine" with the character foundation of integrity, compassion, honesty and wisdom.

[8]This is based on comparative data of health care facilities such as the Geisinger Health Care and Mayo Clinic models (see chap. 12).

[9]Do a web search on "medical doctor salaries" and note the documentation of this point. This is one factor behind the trend for smaller hospitals to merge with other hospitals, according to this information. Presumably the sharing of resources will enhance quality and enable cost savings to stem the transition to new models of financing combined with qualitative and quantitative measurements.

[10]Jonathan Oberlander, "Health Care Policy in an Age of Austerity," *New England Journal of Medicine* 365 (2011): 1075-77.

increased in the United States since then). To use these costly technologies within their frugal health care system, the Japanese medical "power" pressured suppliers to make smart (less costly) MRIs to fit their health care budgets.[11]

In keeping with the corporate and communal character of health care, as well as the historical tradition in which health care was a gratis service of the church, might the formation of local health care cooperatives (in which doctors, nurses and clients all participate in the earnings of the cooperative) pave the way for new models, with financial benefit to all? Here the co-op board might set salaries.

Let's hear the call to justice as an opportunity to love each other in practical ways. Let's hear it as a concrete way of fulfilling Jesus' command to love God with all our heart, soul, mind and strength, and to love our neighbors as ourselves. Further, let's know that healing and peace are ultimately rooted in God and God's gracious gift of life. Healing and shalom reflect God's gracious presence as awesome Creator and loving Parent who redeems us to make justice and truth flourish.

SERVICE

Service is a common word among Christians, but it is in need of rehabilitation. One of the tragic developments in modern American society is the reign of self-absorbed psychology, religion and politics. Robert Bellah, in *Habits of the Heart,* has shown that the historic American value put on individualism has skewed our capacity for social justice and community values.[12] Some church groups, however, have tried to keep alive the vision of the kingdom's call to mission and service. Major renewal of commitment to the welfare of all in the community is desperately needed, whether through the Amish way, a public health insurance option or the controlled low-cost Japanese way.[13] The reign of self-interest and individualism has

---

[11]T. R. Reid, *The Healing of America: A Global Quest for Better, Cheaper, and Fairer Health Care* (New York: Penguin, 2009), p. 84.

[12]Robert Bellah et al., *Habits of the Heart: Individualism and Commitment in American Life* (New York: Harper & Row, 1985), esp. pp. 27-51, 142-63.

[13]Donald Kraybill, Steven M. Nolt and David L. Weaver-Zercher, *The Amish Way: Patient Faith in a Perilous World* (San Francisco: Jossey-Bass, 2010). Is the Amish way of life, with no health insurance but helping each other at all costs, closer to this vision of shalom? I think so, though we may fault them for lack of mission and service. However, the world comes knocking on their door, in literature and travel, to see their serene and simple way of life.

had a huge impact on health care, so that it is no longer a system but an
industry, where market profit drives basic decisions. The concern about *my
rights* leads to many malpractice suits, and that increases health care costs.
While such suits may be justified in view of debilitating health that results
from medical errors, some alternate way of seeking just compensation
might be considered.[14] As it is, the whole society takes on a self-protective
mentality in relation to health insurance and health care. High health
costs and high insurance costs are rooted ultimately in personal fear (see
chap. 6) and lack of communal vision and commitment.

How in the midst of this can we regain an other-directed ethic and
value mission and service as essential aspects of our identity?[15] Can we
regain or maintain a vision for mission and service? If our commitment to
mission and service collapses, so will our interest in health care and our
willingness to fund its accessibility. We will have abandoned our birthright to the Christian tradition we claim.

The results of sharing groups identifying *motivations* for Christian
service among Mennonite health professionals are significant.[16] The range
is striking, as are agreements on certain fundamental points. The highest
number of responses identified Jesus as the example and model servant.
The second highest was the desire to share talents, money and time with
other people, with emphasis on giving one's own time and service to help
others. Another set of responses focused on being constrained by God's
love to help those in need of medical care. Some identified "circumstances"
in life, noting *service* is at the heart of Americanism. Two identified
"service as essential to Christ's gospel" as the chief motivating factor. One
specified "guilt" as a motivating factor: service is an antidote to our self-

[14]In one case of medical oversight leading to more advanced cancer when diagnosed, two people
from our church small group went as advocates who lamented this oversight to the doctor to
request some compensation. In such face-to-face conversation, the doctor agreed to compen-
sate the requested sum, avoiding a suit which would have cost many more health care dollars.
[15]Dr. Glen Miller's experience in serving people in dire health needs with his and his wife's
combined annual income of $2,000 during his first ten years of marriage and medical practice
(1950s and 1960s) is exemplary. He titles a section "I Found That Service Was Pleasure,"
(*Empowering the Patient* [Indianapolis: Dog Ear, 2009], pp. 82-83). Another excellent example is Dr. Margaret Seton, together with her husband, in primary care, as described in her
article "Providing for Those Who Have Too Little," *New England Journal of Medicine* 365
(2011): 1169-71.
[16]This information is based on a workshop I led on this topic in 1993 in a joint meeting of Mennonite Medical and Nursing Associations in Atchison, Kansas.

centeredness, the original sin of selfishness. Another listed "covenant and church responsibility" as the key factor.

In literature more broadly, three prevailing impulses motivate service: duty, personal prestige or self-fulfillment, and humanitarian interests. But none of these is uniquely Christian. Christian servants serve with a belief in a sovereign God who is mending the fallen creation. This sovereign God is working to overcome evil and suffering in this world. Our service is responsive to God's initiative, seeking to restore creation to the health God intended in the good creation. Christian servants also live with hope that God will triumph, knowing suffering and dying are trumped by resurrection hope. Christian service participates in the reconciling work of Jesus Christ. We love because God first loved us in Christ, and we extend Christ's love, peace and healing to others. In Romans 12:2 *service* is worship (liturgy). Service is worshipful response to God. Worship is the deep structure of *Christian* service.

Three biblical motifs inspire and guide our health care vision and vocations:

1. The first motif comes from the creation narrative in Genesis 1: "And God saw everything that he had made, and indeed, it was very good" (Gen 1:31). Psalm 104 and Psalm 148 praise God for the goodness of creation. Health care honors God's good creation. God is the creator: health care providers are coparticipants in sustaining and mending God's good and marvelous creation, though flawed and fallen through human sin. Both health care providers and patients must remember humans are mortal, as Psalm 49 aptly puts it in its recurring refrain: "Mortals cannot abide in their pomp; / they are like the animals that perish." The rich and the poor alike go down to the grave, yet God will ransom the soul of the righteous one (v. 15).

This two-sided emphasis, the goodness of the creation and human mortality, is most important—we flourish like a flower of the field and when the wind blows life fades (Ps 103:15-16). We need not fear death, for in light of Jesus' resurrection, the firstborn from the dead, we are already given eternal life in Jesus Christ (Jn 3:16), and "whether we live or whether we die, we are the Lord's" (Rom 14:8).[17] This awareness can *cure* the fear

---

[17]Even with much literature on "dying well" over the last decades, Allen Verhey critiques patient and doctor efforts to avoid death at all costs. Patient autonomy, together with insurance cover-

component in the health care system, discussed in chapter six.

In this context of knowing human mortality and eternal life, we thank God for the health we have, even when compromised, and we are grateful for health care providers who assist God in healing us from illnesses and provide means of comfort when dying. When we, family members, friends, or victims of violence and natural disaster experience suffering, we know God and the healing community (health care providers and church prayers) are with us and for us. We trust God's promise to walk with us through the valley of the shadow of death (Ps 23).

2. "Love your neighbor as yourself": In the Gospels Jesus cites this text (from Lev 19:18) and links it to the *Shema*, "Hear, O Israel: the LORD is our God, the LORD alone" (Deut 6:4-5). God then commands the covenant people to love the Lord your God with "all your heart, and with all your soul, and with all your might." These two admonitions are Jesus' double love command: love of God and love of neighbor (Mt 22:34-40; Mk 12:28-34; Lk 10:25-28).[18] "Love your neighbor as yourself" is a guiding principle and motivation for health care providers.

3. The third motif in our vision for service comes from Romans 8: awaiting the redemption of our bodies. Health care functions ultimately within an eschatological promise. Though the human body is amazingly intricate and its healthy functioning astounds, yet we know that we live also with frail and dying bodies. Apostle Paul affirms belief in bodily resurrection because God's creation of the body was good. Thus, he says, God will replace the decaying mortal body with a spiritual immortal body at the resurrection (1 Cor 15:35-56; Phil 3:20-21).

We live toward the vision of a new creation, an eternal city come down to earth (Ezek 47; Rev 21:1-5) when our health care agonies in this life are over. In this new city God "will wipe [away] every tear . . . / and crying and pain will be no more" (Rev 21:4). The "glory of God is its light, and its lamp is the [slain, resurrected] Lamb" (Rev 21:23). Flowing

---

age and lack of discerning communities to aid difficult decisions, is largely responsible for what he titles his excellent article, "Still Dying Badly," *Christian Century*, October 19, 2011, pp. 22-27.

[18]See Victor Paul Furnish for extended exposition, in *The Love Command in the New Testament*, rev. ed. (Nashville: Abingdon, 2010). Elsewhere in the New Testament this command is applied in three different contexts: to the relationship of believers to government (Rom 13:8-9), to legalism and libertinism (Gal 5:14), and to partiality within the Christian congregation, that is, treating differently the rich and the poor (Jas 2:8).

out from the city is a river, lined with trees whose leaves bring healing to the nations (Rev 22:2). This is shalom, toward which the best of our health care efforts point.

CONCLUSION

The challenge facing us, as *servants* of God's shalom, is to intentionally bring to our health care ministries these moral priorities: caring faith communities, practice of mutual aid and seeking justice and compassion. These are essential to health, personally and communally. We are servants of God's healing in this world, while we also hope for the consummation of God's glorious new creation. In this tension between the *already* and *not yet* of God's kingdom, yearning for healing and hope often amid illness, we look to the Holy Spirit to hear and take our heart cries to God, our loving Abba (Rom 8:26-27), our heavenly parent yearning for our shalom.

During our journey here on earth, let us show gratitude for the medical care we receive, whether we are poor (and can't pay) or rich (and have full insurance coverage). The grateful spirit, a frequent Pauline command, may be the best cure for the systemic health care illness. Further, such gratitude will be complemented with respect for those who invest their lives to enable us to enjoy the maximal health in our respective situations of living and dying.

> We give thanks to you, O God, and to health care providers
> whose expertise and service aid our health,
> for this and your healing, O God, we exclaim with the psalmist:
>
> > so that my soul may praise you and not be silent.
> > O LORD my God, I will give thanks to you forever. (Ps 30:12)
>
> > O LORD my God, I cried to you for help,
> > and you have healed me. (Ps 30:2)

12

❖

Living Toward
Sustainable Health Care

*What we need is medical care with a community orientation and a spir-
itual dynamic. . . . [W]e need a method to appraise community needs
through soliciting the concerns, opinions and observation of community
members. . . . To minister to the total person's need within the context of
a community requires a multifaceted approach and multidisciplinary
team. A physician, no matter how talented and energetic, cannot do it
all. Nor can we expect to meet all needs by adding professionals; the cost
would be prohibitive. We must incorporate a broad spectrum of personnel
and involve the people of the community themselves. Then we have a
much greater chance for success in improving health.*

Peter A. Boelens,
"Primary Health Care in an Industrialized Country"

In this last chapter I laud the pioneers who not only work toward health
care systems that are sustainable but also respect the goals of cost containment and the motivations of shalom and service.

A *Newsweek* article appearing in late 2009 described an innovative
health care model that promises cost containment and valuing quality for
patients' health care. The model is the Cleveland Clinic. "The clinic's distinctive feature . . . contrast[s] to most other American hospitals, where
doctors are essentially autonomous professionals; at the clinic physicians
work on fixed salaries and yearly contracts."[1] The clinic is at the forefront

---

[1]Jerry Adler and Jeneen Interlandi, "The Hospital That Could Cure Health Care," *Newsweek*,
December 7, 2009, p. 53. Model for change? Yes, if it does its share in care for the poor and
maintains its charitable non-profit status.

of technological procedures for less invasive surgeries, such as repairing "a heart valve with an incision less than an inch long." Dr. Delos M. Cosgrove, a former cardiac surgeon, is president and chief CEO. His goal is not only cost containment but enhancing patients' shalom during their hospital stay. President Obama visited the hospital in July 2009 to learn more about this model that has reduced by nearly 50 percent the average cost of care for clients in their last two years of life below the most expensive hospitals. "Cosgrove told a Senate hearing in June [2009], the clinic's business practices offer a potential model for the American health industry as it strains to bend the ever-rising cost curve."[2] Teamwork among the doctors enables a much lower stock of medical supplies and devices, and eliminates competition for each doctor getting as much from procedures (needed or not) to better their salaries. Ordering procedures to fix something, even though the doctor knows it likely will not help, is too hard to pass up when pay is part of the deal. Such practice runs counter to the values of shalom and service (chap. 11). The *Newsweek* article merits a careful read and discussion by health care professionals, politicians, church groups and others concerned about health care costs.

The Cleveland Clinic, Mayo Clinic and the Geisinger hospital system in eastern Pennsylvania are not alone in the effort to reduce costs and improve quality.

> When Duke University Medical Center set up a disease-management system for congestive heart failure, coordinating the efforts of cardiologists, primary-care doctors, pharmacists, and nurse practitioners, it drove down the cost of treatment 40 percent in a single year, while reducing readmissions and improving outcomes.[3]

The need for revisioning modes of health care and cost containment is imperative—unless we all become Amish! If the U.S. health system is to survive without bankrupting the federal budget, we must make health insurance affordable. Many health insurance premiums increased approximately 30 percent between 2010 and 2011, and in some cases even more. The health care reform initiated under President Obama's administration sets some controls (80 percent of premium revenue allocated to payment of health

---

[2]Ibid.
[3]Ibid, p. 55. Other similar models have begun in the last several years—a total now of seven, at least.

services), but this does not promise to make health care affordable to all (insurance companies can juggle their accounting to fit the formula without *actually* meeting the ratio). We need new thinking and models to forge a future for America's health care industry. We need a system that works for all.

Perhaps it will happen as it did in Taiwan: a conservative (Republican in the United States) president will launch a universal health care program, to both enhance his chance for reelection and "trump" the long-term Democratic agenda. Or, more likely, it may come as it did in Switzerland, a system that continues insurance companies for those who want to pay and receive more care, but also a universal system grounded in moral conviction that *all* need equal access and basic treatment, which in turn enhances "solidarity" (a key Swiss value) in the face of the cultural diversity of the American people.[4]

Health care professionals, church leaders and politicians will find much in T. R. Reid's *Healing of America* that will unhook us from the many misconceptions that currently obstruct any significant universal health care initiatives. The United States spends around 18 percent of its GDP on health care, with all other industrial nations spending less than half that amount (except Switzerland at 11 percent). The United States needs collaborative thinking (leaving political partisanship behind) to find models that solve the irascible problems the present health care industry has loaded onto the economy. Four health care facilities that have reduced costs by 20-30 percent are health care centers (mostly hospitals) in Grand Junction, Colorado; Seattle Group Care with its "Medical Health Care Home" concept and practice; The Everett Clinic (also in Washington); and Sisters of Mercy in Providence, Rhode Island.[5] We need to return to the goals of shalom and service, reflected in the next two models.

---

[4]T. R Reid describes both these models (*The Healing of America* [New York: Penguin, 2009], pp. 164-81).
[5]For documentation see the video "U.S. Health Care: The Good News in American Medicine," http://video.pbs.org/video/2198039605/. In this PBS program (aired at different times regionally during February 2012) T. R. Reid interviews personnel in each of these medical centers. For text introducing this video, see www.pbs.org/programs/us-health-care-good-news/. Reid identified these health care centers from data developed from research by The Dartmouth Atlas Health Care organization (www.dartmouthatlas.org), which since 1971 has tracked medical cost variations in various U.S. regions (www.google.com/search?q=Dartmouth%20 Atlas%20of%20Health%20Care&ie=utf-8&oe=utf-8&aq=t&rls=org.mozilla:en -US:official&client=firefox-a&source=hp&channel=np).

The two narratives that follow represent alternative responses to health care needs. I expect hundreds of similar centers operate in the United States.[6] These are necessary because of the shortcomings of the dominant health care system. As such they are healing "patches" on the larger health care illness. They are similar to relief agencies that respond to global crises, alleviating pain or supplying food and shelter for people uprooted by war and natural disaster. They are necessary, but the need for a better health care system as a whole continues in the United States.

FUNDING-DRIVEN AND VISION-DRIVEN ORGANIZATIONAL HEALTH CARE MODELS

The following consists of an edited speech Dr. James Nelson Gingerich, who leads the Maple City Health Center, Goshen, Indiana, gave at a forum at the Anabaptist Mennonite Biblical Seminary.[7]

A number of years ago I was president of the medical staff at a community hospital. In that capacity I participated in a hospital board strategic planning retreat during which the conversation focused on identifying and exploiting the most profitable sectors of the local medical marketplace. Eventually someone asked, in essence, "Could it be that focusing on exploiting the profitable part of the market might undermine the hospital's stated mission of enhancing the health of the community as a whole?"

The hospital CEO's response was classic: "No margin, no mission," he

---

[6]Atul Gawande describes two such innovative health care clinics headed by creative and courageous physicians: Jeffrey Brenner in Camden, N.J., and Rushika Fernandopulle in Atlantic City, N.J. The Camden, N.J., model was featured on CNN on March 18, 2012, by Fareed Zakaria in a piece titled "The GPS Road Map for Saving Health Care": <http://globalpublic square.blogs.cnn.com/2012/03/19/fareedzakaria-on-savinghealthcare/>. The title of an article by Atul Gawande, "The Hot Spotters: Can We Lower Medical Cost by Giving the Needed Patients Better Care?" (*New Yorker*, January 24, 2011, pp. 41-51), indicates the focus of these efforts to aid the most needy who abuse health care resources (many E.R. visits and addictions). In both cases a caregiver—preferably not a person in health care—mediates between the health care doctors and nurses and the patient. In the Fernandopulle clinic the two physicians, two nurse practitioners, one social worker, one receptionist and eight "health coaches" for the patients meet daily to update pertinent data on all patients first thing in the morning, usually done within a half hour (ibid., p. 48)! The Geisinger Health Care System in northeastern Pennsylvania has a similar intermediary set of personnel that tracks patients and prescribes where, when and how health care is needed.

[7]Used with permission, but with nonexclusive rights. See the fuller story on the history and development of the Center (www.mchcc.com). Publication of this in another book by Herald Press is in process.

intoned. His point was that only after we ensure the hospital's fiscal soundness and well-being do we have the luxury of worrying about our mission. . . . Isn't taking care of the bottom line a condition of pursuing an organization's mission? . . .

In response to the CEO's "No margin, no mission" assertion, I blurted out, "No mission, no mission." . . . I don't think an organization can have it both ways. If we focus on margin, we jeopardize mission. [O]ver the last twenty years . . . I have become more and more convinced there are two kinds of organizations: the vision-driven ones and the funding-driven ones. Faced with decisions, the basic impulse, from which all else flows, is to ask either, does this move make us more . . . profitable? Or, does this move fit with our vision and our mission, our reason for being? Quite apart from the answers we give, our asking of either question sets fundamental direction.

Do we believe in the power of Jesus to free us institutionally from our bondage to the fear of death (see Heb 2:14-15)? Do we need to focus first on institutional survival, or can we trust our organizations' future to God's provision and protection and instead focus on seeking God's reign and its justice?

I'm not opposed to being practical and fiscally responsible. I make budgets and watch bottom lines carefully; I drive a hard bargain when negotiating agreements with laboratories and Medicaid contractors. But whenever I hear community or church leaders advocating a certain course of action because what is at stake is nothing less than the organization's survival—then I see red flags waving. Whenever I hear such appeals, I ask myself, "What is being advocated here, that would not otherwise seem justifiable? What are we being urged to do that is not consonant with this body's mission and identity?"

Twenty years ago, when I was barely thirty, completely green and admittedly idealistic (not to say naive), I began my work with Maple City Health Care Center with a conviction that we could at least explore alternate ways of approaching our engagement in the world, that being engaged in our community as an organization might not constrain our ethic to one of compromise for the sake of responsibility. The vision of the health care center has evolved over these decades, as we have pursued our vision as we understood it. In that pursuit we have experienced new realities and come to understand our past in new ways. . . . [W]e have come to see new possibilities for community.

From the beginning, and coming out of my experiences of and convictions about the church, I approached the work of Maple City Health Care Center as being about creating a space for people in a diverse but largely low-income neighborhood to come together in ways that would bring some measure of healing to us and to our community. The vision was about breaking down barriers—not unlike those that existed between Jews and Gentiles in New Testament times—and fostering a community of wholeness, integration and healing.

Medical care was certainly part of our thinking about healing, but . . . I was also concerned about bringing together people from various backgrounds. At that time the primary diversity in the neighborhood was not ethnic and racial but socioeconomic. Our early vision statement talked about fostering healthy community in our neighborhood by offering integrated primary care medicine in a way that was neighborhood based and community oriented. But we also talked about offering health care that was "single-tiered," about middle-class and lower-class people receiving care side by side, about neighbors . . . support[ing] the neighborhood and our fledgling health care center.

One of our early stories is about a college faculty couple and a young single woman who was homeless and on welfare. The couple and the single woman were expecting babies, and they all participated in the same prenatal group at the health center. We recognized big differences in their expectations for their children, their experience of their pregnancies and in the resources at their disposal. Yet week after week they brought their anticipation, their anxieties. During the group's final session, when their babies were passed around and admired, and they and the other participants ate together, these parents had come to know each other and identify with each other in ways they could not before have imagined.

From the health center's beginning we also had a sense that the integration we were trying to foster in our neighborhood had to be manifest in our staff structure—that if we were going to allow a vision for community to become a reality, we would need to keep focused on that vision and let it guide everything we did. So we were not just concerned about making sure health care was affordable for our patients. We also wanted to make sure all our staff members were receiving a livable wage, and that wage and wealth disparities among our staff were minimized, that benefits were generous and shared, so all could live with a sense of security and of having enough. The importance of making visible in our staff the integration we were seeking for the community was also manifest in that from the day we opened our doors. We not only sought to make services available for Spanish-speaking patients, but also to employ Latinos as part of our staff. . . .

When in board meetings I would talk about preventive care and fostering community, low-income board members would say that the thing they wanted most in a health care center was to have a doctor willing to see their child when she was sick, and to be able to afford to pay the bill.

One low-income board member thought we should accept as patients people in poverty living anywhere in town: "I've got poor friends on the west side of town. Why shouldn't they be able to come here?" We had conversations over a matter of months about whether we wanted to be a health care provider of last resort, only taking care of poor people, or whether we, having located our center in the town's lowest income neighborhood, wanted to serve that neighborhood as a whole, regardless of residents' income. Did we want to be the place people came because they had no alternative, or did we want to be an integral part of a neighborhood? Did we want to be an organization people could feel good about belonging to, because here we work together to build strong community organizations: a great elementary school, for example, and lively churches, and a health care center for the whole neighborhood? Did we want to be a resource the community could take ownership in, or would we be a place where only the desperate sought help? . . .

Early on, we developed the sense that we exist to serve a vision for community. We wanted that vision to guide everything we did, not just in developing program, but in determining the funding we would seek, how we would structure and recruit staff, and how the staff and board would function. Vision was central, and in our decision-making discussions, an appeal to vision was a trump card anyone could play. On the other hand, any argument that we needed to set aside vision for the sake of survival, in order to avoid financial risk or enhance our solvency, would be suspect immediately. We would not compromise vision for matters of practicability.

A new era in thinking about our vision occurred in the mid-1990s when I was invited to attend a Healthy Communities Summit in San Francisco. It was my first sustained exposure to asset-based community development. Those who adopt this approach focus not on a community's problems but on its assets. They foster and build on the gifts and strengths already present in a community. As John McKnight has written, "Care is . . . the manifestation of a community. The community is the site for the relationship of citizens. And it is at this site that the primary work of the caring society must occur. If that site is invaded, co-opted, overwhelmed and dominated by service-producing institutions, then the work of community will fail." This approach raised the question: How can we foster becoming a site for relationship among neighbors rather than being a service-producing institution? . . .

My learning [from the conference] fit with where we'd already been, but it consolidated directions and gave us ways of talking about these priorities. In deciding to focus on the neighborhood instead of just poor people we had already been thinking about how we could be an asset for the community, not merely a place for the desperate to bring their problems. We had had a history in fostering groups (like our mom-to-mom program) that connected people and helped them be less isolated. We had already been recruiting staff for their vision and commitments, not just for their competence in doing certain tasks. We had already been thinking imaginatively "outside the box" both as staff and board. But the language of asset-based community development—with its emphasis on building on the gifts and strengths in our community, in our staff, in our relationships—provided a vocabulary for thinking and talking about our work, and helped us refocus with new clarity. . . .

As a health center staff, we had been trying to address the isolation of some members of our community by identifying activities they enjoy and inviting patients who enjoy similar activities to do them together. We had identified some people who enjoy cooking, and had invited them to meet in the health center's community room on Wednesday afternoons to cook for each other. Some people in the group spoke English and some spoke Spanish, and they were beginning to learn each other's language as they enjoyed each other's food.

Half a dozen years ago I attended a Mennonite Health Assembly meeting which featured Doug Eby, a Mennonite physician who led a restructuring of Native American health services in Alaska. Over about a dozen years he helped transform that system from a typical bureaucratic clinic structure, organized around medical providers, into a Native owned and operated system of care. One result was a huge improvement in patient access. But Eby says, *"It's not about access.* Access is only a tool that helps create relationships because it breaks down barriers. Relationships are really what it's all about. It is only through solid relationships that you can begin to get at insidious underlying health issues such as depression, domestic violence, and obesity."

Through our exposure to Doug Eby's story we found a straightforward approach to discernment about what we are trying to do by asking three questions:

1. Does it foster long-term relationships?
2. Does it increase integration? And
3. Does it empower people?

These themes of relationship-based care, integration, and empowerment were already present in our approach, but this new shorthand gave us a tool to use more consistently and more broadly. We began explicitly asking these questions of all programmatic initiatives, of all funding initiatives, of all policy proposals. We even restructured our employee evaluations around these questions.

1. What about your job fosters long-term relationships with patients, with other staff, with members of the community? And what about your job gets in the way of such relationships?
2. What about your job fosters integration of care for patients? Your integration with the staff into the community? Your personal integration (job and rest of life)? And what about your job gets in the way of such integration?
3. What about your job is empowering for you? Empowering for others? What about your job is disempowering?

Now we use these same three questions to evaluate everything we do. In itself this evaluative tool becomes a new locus of integration. Over time we have observed that administrative staff that spend too much time in their offices and lack significant direct interaction with patients don't feel adequately fed by their work, and they eventually burn out and leave. And so we have developed an organizational principle that all staff should have direct patient contact in the regular course of their work.

Another point Doug Eby made that has become transformative for us is his call to escape the "tyranny of the traditional physician-patient encounter." This one-on-one, private, behind-closed-doors encounter, characterized by huge power differentials, is about as non-conducive a set-up for building community as one could find. It does not tend to foster authentic long-term relationships, it does not tend to empower patients, and it is therefore unlikely to foster integration between medical encounter and needed lifestyle changes or other aspects of daily life.

So we began to explore more intentionally models for providing health care in groups. We had groups in various settings before: prenatal classes, mom-to-mom groups, support groups for survivors of sexual abuse, the cooking and eating group, get-togethers for coffee. And our board meetings and staff meetings were group activities. But all these were on the margins of the health care we offer. We had never tried to address health care itself in a group model.

So our steps to begin group care at the health care center did not stem from an effort to be more cost-effective, or more efficient in using staff time, but rather directly out of a challenge to reconfigure our structures to enhance relationships, integration, and empowerment.

We started our group efforts in two areas. First we explored an approach to prenatal care called Centering Pregnancy, a model developed initially at Yale midwifery school and refined over more than a decade. Here 6-10 pregnant women, whose babies are due at about the same time, meet together 8 times. During the two-hour gatherings, one of their health care providers (physician or midwife) is present. We meet in the living room of a little yellow bungalow next door to the health center. The first half hour we spend measuring each woman's belly, while the others weigh themselves, check their blood pressures, and help themselves to a glass of juice or water and fruit and crackers. Then we spend an hour and a half all together in a circle (some women also bring their partners), talking about the things in this pregnancy that are important to them. The role of staff is not to teach or bring expert opinion to bear on every question, but to facilitate participation of all the members of the group, and help the women see how much they bring to the group from their own experience and background.

We've learned to ask open-ended questions. I used to ask, "Are you planning to breastfeed?" The right answer was clear, and if someone ventured to say no, I had lost them for possible breastfeeding. Now we typically ask something like, "What have you been thinking about feeding your baby?" or even "What have you heard or thought about breastfeeding?" . . .

In the course of these groups, not only does medical care happen, not only is there lots of education in a context that affirms what they know and have learned, but in the course of the twenty hours they spend together, these women form a supportive network of relationship. Especially our Latina patients, who in Mexico would experience pregnancy and childbirth surrounded by mother, grandmothers, sisters, and aunts, often find themselves isolated in Goshen, perhaps with a partner as their only support. Centering groups soon became places for significant friendship and support.

So we started these Centering Pregnancy groups and immediately had a strong sense of their potential. We had hired Beth, a midwife with extensive previous experience with this approach to prenatal care, and the groups were wonderful. Initially we conducted some groups in English, and some in Spanish. Not only did our prenatal patients attend with regularity, but staff came from these groups excited and energized by the interaction and by what we were learning.

But soon we found we did not have enough pregnant English-speaking patients to offer English-only groups. So we decided to try to have bilingual groups, with everything being interpreted both ways. As far as we knew, no one had tried this approach in Centering Pregnancy groups, and we were afraid that all the bilingual interpreting might be cumbersome and ungainly.

But we also saw the potential for cross-cultural bridge-building, and the development of new relationships. I started the first bilingual group by observing that the Anglos and Hispanics in our town have few opportunities to get to know each other, but the children we are preparing for will likely play with each other, go to school with each other, and may eventually start new families together. So as we prepare for these children, we also want to prepare a shared community to receive them.

We were surprised to discover that the discipline of interpreting everything into English and Spanish, far from being awkward and intrusive, helped us listen better. People can only speak about one breath's worth, one or two sentences, before they need to wait for translation. And only one person can speak at a time. So people speak with greater care, and listen more carefully. . . .

Maple City Health Care Center relies on grants to meet about fifteen percent of our budget; the rest is provided by contributions (ten percent) and fees for service (seventy-five percent). Because we are committed to having vision rather than have funding drive our work, we don't ask the question, "What grants can we apply for, for which we can meet the funding entity's objectives?" Instead we ask, "What are we already doing or planning to do, that we can describe in such a way that a funding agency will recognize it as something they want to support?" It is rare that we find grant applications inspiring, let alone that they transform what we do.

But one day I was writing a grant application and came to the question, "How does your board reflect the diversity of your patient population?" I gulped. "It doesn't" didn't seem like a promising answer. It wasn't that we didn't want lower-income and non-Anglo members on our board. We did. We had asked a variety of people to serve on our board. When the health care center was forming a decade and a half earlier, we had gathered community leaders of various classes and subcultures to form a board: the principal of the elementary school across the street and some parents of children attending the school, a family physician, a lawyer, a nurse living in the neighborhood, a school social worker, tenants working with a community organization to create rental housing standards, people working in local factories. As we generated ideas, made plans, raised funds, and rehabbed a building, there were plenty of ways for all kinds of people to get involved and contribute.

As the years went by, though, the work of the board became a matter of gathering for monthly meetings to oversee operations, approve budgets, establish policies—in short, middle-class institutional agenda. Looking back, I began to realize that what we had tried was a classic approach to board function that relied on middle-class white assumptions about how you do business. You develop an agenda and you proceed through it in an orderly fashion, discussing each item and making decisions where necessary. The non-middle-class members had been committed enough to the health care center that they hung in there for a while with a board organization and process that was foreign to them, but eventually they drifted away.

What else could we do? . . . At that point, we had a board composed of six middle-class Anglos, ranging in age from forty-something to ninety-something. The board included two staff members, Beth (our nurse midwife) and me. All the board members are wonderful people, deeply committed to the organization, and most had served on the board for ten years or longer. . . . Beth and I proposed that we experiment with borrowing from the Centering Pregnancy circle model of group interaction and facilitative leadership, especially as we had adapted the model to cross-cultural groups. For months the board had been hearing the staff's excitement about the Centering Pregnancy groups, and they responded to the proposal without hesitation: "We have so much to gain and nothing to lose. Let's go for it."

We decided to invite four people to join a reconstituted board. All four were patients, and we selected them after inviting our whole staff to consider the question, "Who of our patients is deeply involved in the life of our neighborhood and brings passion and energy to their interactions at the health care center?" The four staff people recommended were an Anglo single mother of seven, a factory worker who had been involved in student organizing as a youth in Mexico City, an employed Latina mother of two who had participated in a Centering Pregnancy group, and another young Latina mother.

In order to include everyone, we needed to function differently. We gave up our typical middle-class agenda-driven meetings and instead started each meeting with an extended conversation around the circle that began with a question that helps us think about how we relate to our community. A meeting might begin with: "Tell us about what it is like to be a longtime resident (or a new immigrant) in this community? Where do you feel connected? Isolated? Alienated?" Or the leader might ask, "What has been your experience with medical care in our community? Elsewhere?" All our conversations take place at table, around good food, and they are blessed by the deliberate pace enforced by English-Spanish and Spanish-English interpretation. Translating content is important, but even more essential is the time we take to speak and listen carefully. . . .

We try to stay within our two-hour time limit for meetings, but invariably people stick around for awhile to help with dishes, or just to chat. One board member told us not long ago, "This is the most civilized part of my life. At work I'm in the jungle. Here we listen." Several members have remarked that nowhere else do they interact at such depth with people whose experiences and perspectives are so different from their own.

We are now three years into this way of conducting board meetings. And every month I go into our meetings weary after a long day in the office—and leave with a renewed sense that this is the most exciting and satisfying work I could possibly do.

All of us are familiar with the "progression" from idealistic initiative to the inexorable bureaucratic processes of institutions. We even accept as necessary a certain organizational "maturation," like the one Max Weber has famously described, from the charismatic to the bureaucratic. I wonder whether that progression doesn't coincide with, or develop out of, a shift from initial clarity of purpose to a focus on institutional survival. That shift I believe is deadly to our imagination and consigns us to a kind of living death.

If we want to avoid that kind of dying, I think we need to name our fear of death and attendant focus on survival as temptations from which we daily pray to be delivered. When we start talking about being realistic, practical, and responsible, we need to consider whether we are moving away from dependence on God and trying instead to secure our own future. We need to recognize and name as seductive that siren song of survival, and listen to those who question where it calls us to go.

I have drawn these alternatives starkly in order to clarify what I think are the dangers. But I believe that any organization that wants to draw its inspiration from and orient its future toward a vision of a new reality needs to encourage and bless those who can help us stay focused on that vision. We need to heed those who invite us to be imaginative about our strengths and resources and possibilities, however insufficient they seem. Then, if my experience is any gauge, we will watch those possibilities multiply and re-joice in the abundance God provides.

[Note: Reported in local newspapers in mid-August 2009 the Center recently began a "Community Service for Pay" program, for those who cannot pay, because of unem-ployment. Their medical bills are reduced or paid completely by doing community service.]

Work as Worship, Prayer and Healing

The following stories come from Dr. Tim Leaman, who is associate medical director of Esperanza Health Center in Philadelphia, founded in 1989. Dr. Leaman's article begins with his reflection on Psalm 114:7-8. The central motif in his article is how hard rock becomes springs of living water: living in hope. He juxtaposes his meditation with recounting "yes-terday's" encounter with five patients and the dire situations of their lives. I select one to illustrate how a pray-er at the clinic can be part of the healing process. Then his article moves to how our work can be worship, how worship sustains our work, and our work returns to the one we worship. From this part I report only "Pablo's story" to exemplify holistic health, including the spiritual dimension of one's life.

Yesterday at the clinic. I sat with a woman who had only weeks before moved from Puerto Rico, where she was leaving an abusive relationship with a live-in boyfriend who had recently begun to use drugs again. She left her three-year-old son there with him. She brought a ten-year-old and a six-year-old son with her (the younger of which is severely behaviorally challenged, likely because of the crack his mother used while he was in utero). Now she just had to move out from the friend [and children] she had been staying with here, because they couldn't tolerate her son's out-of-control behavior. She had been part of a church in Puerto Rico in her past, and had made a break from her previous crack addiction, but wasn't connected to any supports here. She had no job, no place to stay, no family here, no church. She just started smoking four days ago, after six years stopped, because she feels so overwhelmed. She started to cry when I began to share about the possibility of reconnecting to God. She was eager when I offered that one of our medical assistants could pray with her, and she took the name of a church I recommended near where she was staying.[8]

Pablo's story. "He took away my manhood," spilled out this 60-year old man just before breaking into tears on his first visit to our office, as he shared his story of an unsuccessful surgery, now almost 15 years ago. He was squeezed into the final walk-in slot of the day, and I recognized quickly that this would be a challenging visit.

The story poured out in desperate bursts and fragments—from the old surgery, to the "fire" that still burned in his stomach. A decade and a half before, he had begun to have a significant abdominal pain and a surgeon in the Chicago area attempted unsuccessfully to correct it. The aftermath was severe post-surgical complications resulting in a long hospital stay, and later two repeat surgeries to attempt to resolve the problem. But the three surgeries, rather than solving anything, left him in worse pain than ever.

"I lost everything," he said, as he described how his inability to work led to the loss of his job, the disintegration of his marriage and the onset of deep depression. Now, years later, after several moves and many doctors, he continued to have severe chronic abdominal pain, which hadn't been controlled.

"He ruined my life," he repeated over and over as he relayed the story, between spells of tears. His angry tone suggested that now bitterness as much as pain controlled his life.

[8]Tim Leaman, "Hard Rock into Springs of Water: Working in Hope." *Mennonite Health Journal* 11, no. 3 (2009): 9.

When I gently raised this observation, he didn't disagree, rather going on to explain the preoccupation he has lived with of gaining revenge on this surgeon. He had finally left the Chicago area at least partly because of his recurring urge to find this man and kill him. Now distance was between them, but the hatred still burned.

Unsure what to offer, I asked, "Are you part of any church or religious background?" And immediately the tears began to flow again and a whole new story unfolded.

He had been active in ministry in a church in Chicago, even traveling as part of evangelistic campaigns in Latin America, together with holding a well-paying job there before all these medical complications struck.

Together with everything else, his ministry had crumpled. He had continued to attend church and had attended a Pentecostal congregation in the year since he had moved to Philadelphia, but he continued to struggle mightily with why God had allowed all this to happen in his life.

Renewing Pablo's expired depression medicines and anti-acid medicines, along with referring him to a stomach specialist, was an easy place to start. As it was already late and we had long since passed our scheduled time for the visit, I considered delaying any further interventions until a follow-up visit could be arranged. What more could be done, anyway, in a few short minutes for pains that had obviously been years in the making? I wondered.

But a clear inner tugging pushed me further. "I want you to restart these medicines," I said, "but I really think that's only dealing with a piece of your problem."

Knowing I was venturing out on a limb, but feeling a boldness rising up within, I shared, "It's clear this condition has taken over your life. The bitterness you feel toward this surgeon is consuming you. Unless you begin to release your hatred to this surgeon, I don't think you're ever going to be able to move forward. And I doubt we'll be able to treat your stomach pain."

I didn't know what to expect. But as we continued to share, it seemed that something had struck a chord.

"Can we pray for you," I asked, "that God would touch the places you're hurting and help you to let go of this bitterness?" Pablo readily agreed. And so we prayed together for healing, for grace to forgive, for freedom and for God's love to be felt in Pablo's heart.

A few weeks later, I got a letter from the gastroenterologist and pictures from Pablo's stomach. He had seen some active inflammation and agreed with continuing the anti-acid medicine.

Not long after that, Pablo returned for his follow-up visit. As the medical assistant brought him toward a room, he cheerily stopped to shake my hand and greet me warmly. As I entered the room, it was evident something had changed. No sooner had I sat down, than he declared, "I'm a whole new person!"

"Ever since we prayed together," he continued, "things are different. I've started praying for my surgeon. I forgave him and now I'm praying for his salvation. I've been able to worship again. I've felt peace. My stomach pain is gone. I talked to my pastor and there might be opportunities for me to start serving in our church. I'm a completely different person."

As Pablo thanked me repeatedly, I listened in amazement, remembering how close I'd come to sending him home with just a few pills. Yet somehow God had used a small step of faith to bring a radical transformation in his heart and body. And the same medicines that had failed to control the pain previously now were working perfectly—the extra acid of bitterness apparently forgiven away.

"God is so wonderful," gushed Pablo. I couldn't agree more.[9]

---

[9]Ibid., pp. 24-25.

Summary and
Concluding Reflections

The three parts of this book are hinged together by the book's title, *Health, Healing, and the Church's Mission: Biblical Perspectives and Moral Priorities.* The subtitle also charts the course of the contribution of the book: stronger in the first parts on biblical perspectives and then stronger on moral priorities in the last part. But the interplay between the two accents of the subtitle must be emphasized. Every aspect of the biblical perspective explicitly or implicitly consists also of a moral dimension. The moral accent of chapters ten to twelve is deeply embedded in the biblical perspective. The church's mission is defined and empowered by both dimensions.

Seven theses, the united Old Testament and New Testament witness to God/Jesus Christ/Holy Spirit as Healer, the four paradoxes, and the church's response in healing ministry delineate the first part and foundation of the book's contribution. Of special note are the impact of God's good creation with God's desire for human shalom (which includes holistic health) and the effect of the Fall that fights against God's purposes. It is precisely in this tension between these two theological and human realities that God/Jesus Christ/Holy Spirit is healing promise, both in the now and not yet. Within this tension falls also the human experience of shalom and sickness; living and dying; God's eternity and human mortality; God's healing work in the world and Satan's obstructions through divisions, arrogance, violence and war, which exacerbate sickness and disease (note, e.g., the plight of injured war veterans) and frustrate God's and the church's healing mission.

Because of God's good creation and this "other" reality that fights against that goodness the theodicy problem looms large. How does one affirm belief in this good, healing God in the face of suffering that insidiously marks the human experience, whether that suffering comes from human error, accidents, the dying process, natural calamity, genetic factors or inexplicable causes? We cannot say God wills this, but we can say God is with and for us in our suffering (chap. 4). When children are afflicted with suffering, such as handicaps or cancer, the struggle to affirm God's healing presence is even harder, yet all the more necessary.

The church's mission includes embodying the divine healing presence and embrace that prays, helps and encourages in such situations. And all the time, in the midst of striving for genuine Christian community, we pray for healing, even miracles, knowing that God is gracious, and will on occasion bring the promised complete healing of the eschaton into our present experience. In all this is both mystery and cause for praise. When healing happens, through medical or divine achievement, our best response is: "so that my soul may praise you and not be silent. O LORD my God, I will give thanks to you forever" (Ps 30:12).

Three issues from part one of this book merit notice in this summary. First, though God intends shalom for human experience, shalom and health cannot be equated (recall the too-broad, encompassing WHO definition of health). For many of us, illness of one sort or another marks our life. While this at times interrupts shalom, it does not negate it. Nor does it silence praise of God. Shalom comes in following God's calling for our lives, though risks in that calling may cause illness, even death. Faithfulness to the calling and trust in God/Jesus are more important than health. For this, witness the lives of missionaries—Schweitzer and Livingstone, for example. Health can become an idol, as modern life with its medical expertise is prone. Even in illness, we can experience shalom as God's gift.

Second, in the New Testament especially, suffering and human weakness mark Christian experience. God's resurrection power shines through the *cross*. For Paul, his strength is made perfect in his weakness, that is, "power is made perfect in weakness" (2 Cor 12:9). This is said precisely in the context of Paul's asking God three times to take away his affliction, but God did not (for the larger theological point, see 2 Cor 4:7-12; 13:4). Thus suffering ought not—does not—close us to God's working in our lives, nor to our praise of God. Rather, because of this basic paradox running from Job; to Isaiah, servant of the Lord; to Jesus; to Paul, suffering and persecution becomes a mark of the faithful (1 Thess 1:6-7; Col 1:24; Rev). As Gaiser puts it, "Healing in Christ is ultimately cruciform (e.g. Isa. 53:5; Luke 23:35; Acts 3:15-16; 2 Cor. 12:5-10)."[1]

Third, what is the role of faith in healing? The Gospel narratives often, but not always, mention faith as a positive factor—even condition—for healing. This faith is directed, however, to Jesus as One sent by God, God's Son bringing healing and salvation. Salvation is linked to healing in the New Testament: the one word *sōzō* can be translated either as "heal" or "save." Faith then plays a broader role than only to obtain physical healing; it orients one passionately to the saving Christ. Hence healings are often, then and now in mission work, linked to people coming to salvation, and praising God/Jesus as Savior.

Further, when the healing we pray for does not happen as we want, this is not to be taken as reason to condemn oneself or others for lack of faith. Healing is always God's/Jesus' gift; it is not *our* faith or doing. And when we are not healed from physical sickness as we might desire, we may experience other dimensions of healing, emotional and spiritual, and know shalom-joy even when health is compromised. The healing psalms remind us of just this point. The complaint psalms usually turn to praise, even though aching bones and eyes tearing with grief do not end. Even in those psalms, like 86, which I read this morning, the supplicant affirms the steadfast love and faithfulness of the Lord (Ps 86:5, 13, 15).

As churches commit themselves to ministries of healing it is important to keep these three emphases in mind.

The middle section of this book addresses both the biblical foundation of the church's health care mission and narrates this mission historically. Justice, shalom, mutual sharing and care for the disabled are primary emphases. The church's healing work (chap. 5) is extended theologically and practically in chapters six through nine. Mutual aid and care for one another mark the church's paradigm for health care through the ages and into our modern context. As Christians we must resist the temptation to

---

[1]Frederick J. Gaiser, *Healing in the Bible* (Grand Rapids: Baker Academic, 2010), pp. 245-50. (For his summary of this scope of biblical teaching see his points 1, 2, 6, 11, 12, 16, 17, 21, 26, 27, 30.) His summary is mostly applicable to my work as well.

look to modern economics and medical expertise for our moral answer to the issues that plague us in current health care debates. Rather, Christians must bring the wider and deeper theological and moral perspective to these debates, founded on Scripture and the historic mission of the church in healing and health care.

For the health care portion of this book, it is important to recognize that providing health insurance for all is important and daunting, but not necessarily an imperative task (remember the Amish). Caring for the sick requires much more than insurance. It means compassionate presence; pastoral visitation of the sick incarnates gospel hope: healing, recovery, health and life—but if not, in the end God.[2] Compassionate presence is essential for care of the disabled. But it is not only *for* them; it is really *with* them, so that in community we learn the grace of mutual care. *Mutual care and aid* is more than (really, other than) health insurance. At this juncture in Christian history, only communities like the Amish, the Hutterites and small new monastic communities truly practice mutual aid. Just as the Amish reflexively practice forgiveness, as the stories in *Amish Grace* attest,[3] so they also practice mutual aid to pay their health care costs.[4] Anabaptist-Mennonite self-defined organizations provide a mix of health insurance and mutual aid, a model that represents what numerous other denominations have done as well, to lesser or greater degrees. This mix creates a challenge to how we respond to those who cannot afford health insurance and to moral clarity on the relation of health insurance to mutual aid.

We live in a time when change is coming to health care in the United States. Whatever health care reform does or does not develop in the next decade, the industry's delivery systems and costs will continue to challenge the sustainability of the United States' health care system. A competitive health care market with various players likely will continue (see chap. 10). This means the complex health care system will continue, with market profit for all the players in the industry. Whether overall costs can be contained—or, better, reduced—remains an open question. What moral

---

[2]Cf. Philip H. Pfatteicher, "Some Early and Later Fathers on the Visitation of the Sick," *Pro Ecclesia* 19, no. 2 (2010): 213-14.

[3]Donald B. Kraybill, Steven M. Nolt and David L. Weaver-Zercher, *Amish Grace: How Forgiveness Transcended Tragedy* (San Francisco: Jossey-Bass, 2007).

[4]Donald B. Kraybill, Steven M. Nolt and David L. Weaver-Zercher, *The Amish Way: Patient Faith in a Perilous World* (San Francisco: Jossey-Bass, 2010).

responsibility do we as Christians have to care for the health needs of those in our churches and for others also? With *profit* the tail that wags the health care dog (or should the image be reversed?), Mary McDonough has rightly raised the question, "Can a health care market be moral?"[5]

Many Christians who work in the health professions struggle with the challenge of how to hold together their Christian motivations for their vocation with the legal and competitive business demands of their profession. The essays in *The Changing Face of Health Care* document and illustrate through specific quandaries the complexity that health professionals deal with.[6] It is sad when a competent nurse says, "Almost daily, I have to lie to insurance companies to get what the patient needs."[7] Or as Vicki, a "competent and compassionate rehabilitation nurse," says, "I find that the changes in health care have impacted the personalization of nursing. There is decreased time to spend with the patient's emotional needs."[8]

The challenge to hold fast to Christian values and not to become discouraged faces health professionals at all levels, whether at the Menninger psychiatric hospital, the Mayo Clinic or the local doctor's office. Volunteer time by doctors, nurses, social workers and others in low-cost or free clinics for those who have no insurance and perhaps cannot pay is a witness to the ethic of the Christian gospel. May these continue and flourish as the lifeboat for those who otherwise would drown and as a lighthouse for those in health care professions who can no longer find a moral alternative to the system in which they, of necessity, practice. We live at a time when new initiatives at the federal level may generate hope that the disparity in health care access between the rich and poor may be overcome, in part at least. But the political resistance, largely to protect the wealthy—who finance the election campaigns of the lawmakers—at the expense of the poor and lower middle class, looms large also.

In constructing new facilities and developing new technologies, we must ask, are the available resources already enough for this area? Is it

[5]Mary J. McDonough, *Can a Health Care Market Be Moral? A Catholic Vision* (Washington, D.C.: Georgetown University Press, 2007). Compare Allen Verhey's chapter, "Can Medical Ethics Be Christian?" in *Theological Voices in Medical Ethics*, ed. Allen Verhey and Stephen Lammers (Grand Rapids: Eerdmans, 1993), pp. 30-56.
[6]John F. Kilner, Robert D. Orr and Judith Allen Shelly, ed., *The Changing Face of Health Care* (Grand Rapids: Eerdmans, 1998).
[7]Barbara J. White, "A Nurse's Experience," in ibid., p. 22.
[8]Ibid., p. 20.

ethical, by any standard, to duplicate high-tech medical equipment within a small city or town population when many parts of our own country, let alone less technologically advanced countries, don't have even one specialist or a given technology (e.g., MRI) within a one- or two-hour drive? In 1992 I witnessed the first day's use of an MRI in a small hospital of high repute in Taiwan. How many cities or hospitals in the world still don't have even one MRI? When does more equal distribution of expensive resources take precedence over the desire to expand one's own technology when the same is available within a one- to ten-mile drive? These, and similar issues, need our moral scrutiny and compassionate wisdom. It may be, as Jacob Weisberg writes in his review of T. R. Reid's *Healing of America*, that America's health care system will always be more costly than that of any other nation, since every nation's health care system is unique to and reflective of its culture. America's will be a "uniquely American solution," costly, to be sure, to reflect our culture.[9] But nonetheless, the present system/industry must change, for it is economically unsustainable and morally bankrupt.

In the last half century many new hospitals developed, especially as mission and service arms of the Catholic and Methodist churches, and other denominations as well. The last half century also has seen an ever-increasing effort to provide more patient-oriented health care. Many young men and women entered into medicine, nursing and related health fields out of commitment to serve fellow humanity. One of the planks in the present health care reform effort is to improve health care for the patient by moving from "procedure" billing and payment to reward for quality patient care.

An anomaly of our time is the disjunction between supporting health care missions overseas and yet resisting improvement of the United States' broken health care system, so as to provide affordable health care access for all citizens. Health care access is a moral issue of shalom, compassion, mission and service, whether that be provided through religious bodies, federal or state initiatives, insurance companies, or community mutual aid (the Amish and the Hutterites). Another anomaly is resistance to health care initiatives because of opposition to government interference and

---

[9]Jacob Weisberg, "We Are What We Treat: Fixing Health Care, American Style," *Newsweek*, July 27, 2009, p. 27.

funding. Yet most critics who oppose health care reforms have no qualms about accepting federally funded Social Security, Medicare, Medicaid, Veterans' or other health care benefits when eligible to receive them.

If the church would follow the imperative of the parable of the good Samaritan, the church would humbly and eagerly fulfill its mission in health care, at home and abroad, and not only for its own or to protect the wealthy. We need historical perspective on health care, with gratitude for the good that church and government have done in the past and continue to do in the present to make health care a benefit many Americans receive cheerfully.

Facing these dilemmas and new challenges, let us keep the biblical and historical mandates in mind. However the future unfolds, we are implored not to forget the model of the early Christian church, to care for one another as God has cared for us in the mutual gift of the Father, Son and Spirit for our salvation and healing, now and in the life to come.

> I owe the Lord a morning song
>   of gratitude and praise,
> for the kind mercy he has shown
>   in lengthening out my days.
> He kept me safe another night;
>   I see another day.
> Now may his Spirit, as the light,
>   direct me in his way.[10]

---

[10]Amos Herr, "I Owe the Lord a Morning Song" (1890).

APPENDIX 1

————❖————

Mennonites, Brethren and Related Groups in Health Care

In his article on the Anabaptist tradition in *Caring and Curing*, Walter Klaassen identifies the visible peoplehood of God in the congregation as the context and basis for all thinking about health care in the church.

> Their church was a visible, concrete certainty, in which members became brothers and sisters in the family of God, welded together in obedience and in faithfulness with their elder brother, Jesus. . . .
>
> Membership in this caring family of God brought with it the gift of well-being—insofar as this is attainable in this world. . . . The chief characteristic of well-being was *gelassenheit*, . . . the abandonment of self-will and nonresistant surrender to the will of God.[1]

Klaassen describes the origin and development of Mennonite health care endeavors, be it the traveling preacher-physician, as was common in the Netherlands, the office and work of ordained deaconesses, which prevailed among Mennonites until 1950, or the formation of numerous Mennonite health societies, which in some cases contracted with a local physician for a monthly fee to provide for health care needs for all in the Mennonite community (most notably the Mennonite Health Society in Coaldale, Alberta, begun in 1928). From this same sense of peoplehood and care for each other as brothers and sisters, mutual aid agencies developed in the Mennonite Church in local regions and in the organization,

---

[1]Walter Klaassen, "The Anabaptist Tradition," in *Caring and Curing: Health and Medicine in the Western Religious Traditions*, ed. Ronald L. Numbers and Darrel W. Amundsen (New York: Macmillan, 1986), pp. 273-74.

Mennonite Mutual Aid Association (now Everence).

In his foreword to Graydon Snyder's book *Health and Medicine in the Anabaptist Tradition*, Martin Marty begins by quoting 1 Corinthians 1:28 and then describes Anabaptist health care practices as "countercultural because their approach to understandings of health and illness, care and cure, groping for meaning and coping with suffering and death, is communal."[2] Of the four social science grids of Mary Douglas and Bruce Malina, Snyder classifies the Anabaptist types as "low individualism-high community."[3] Snyder's book is a rich read. Already in 1663 Prussian Mennonites organized a fire insurance association, and this type of mutual aid/insurance approach dominated twentieth-century Anabaptist-descended groups in the United States.[4] Snyder also notes that other helping groups reflect high communal commitment, such as Alcoholics Anonymous, twelve-step programs, and base communities in Central and South America. They are there for each other, to encourage and inspire, to help and to care. These new communitarians may be the Anabaptists of the twenty-first century, as those historically Anabaptist groups become more acculturated, attuned to dominant American culture.[5] The *caring* of these communities is rooted in mutual aid, Christ and service, and mutual (covenant) love.[6]

From these communities such agencies emerged as the Heifer Project, Church World Service, Mennonite Central Committee, Ten Thousand Villages (selling handicrafts made in poor countries worldwide) and Howard Zehr's creative work in victim-offender reconciliation programs.[7] Chris Marshall, Anabaptist Mennonite Biblical Seminary graduate in the seminary's master of peace studies, with a prior Ph.D. in New Testament, initiated such reconciliation programs in New Zealand with biblical and theological interpretation. Princess Anne (U.K.) presented an award to him for his outstanding ministry.

Coupled with this "Christ and service" motivation, numerous mission programs emerged, often combining gospel teaching and evangelism with

---

[2] Martin Marty, foreword to Graydon Snyder's *Health and Medicine in the Anabaptist Tradition* (Valley Forge: Penn.: Trinity Press International, 1995), pp. ix, xi.
[3] Snyder, *Health and Medicine*, p. 21.
[4] Ibid.
[5] Ibid., pp. 78, 120-23.
[6] Ibid., pp. 73-81.
[7] Howard Zehr, *Changing Lenses: A New Focus for Crime and Justice* (Scottdale, Penn.: Herald Press, 2005).

health care. Between 1851 and 1969 eighty-eight new missions were founded overseas by Mennonite and Brethren in Christ denominations. Of these, at least twenty-eight included medical workers. The bulk of them would have had both doctors and nurses, but in a number of cases the mission included nurses only. They operated clinics for treating patients. Many of the hospitals begun in various countries during the twentieth century are now leading medical training centers, with local citizens heading the medical colleges. What began as low key and informal mushroomed over the years to become major health contributions to a country's health care system.

When the Mennonite Church denomination in North America decided to begin overseas mission work, the first person approved to go overseas as a missionary was medical doctor W. B. Page, from Middlebury, Indiana. However, the board would not send him until a minister could accompany him. In 1899, Dr. Page, Mrs. Page and their young daughter, along with Jacob Ressler, a widower, minister and bishop from Scottdale, Pennsylvania, were sent together to India. They were the first Mennonite missionaries of the Mennonite Church sent overseas from North America.[8]

In a history of Mennonite missions, Wilbert Shenk lists 159 overseas mission programs begun by Mennonite groups from 1850-1999.[9] Health care of some type was a significant aspect of many of the mission initiatives. One distinctive feature of the earlier period was that women, trained in the United States as medical doctors, were not yet accepted in the United States but flourished in their medical ministry overseas (e.g., Florence Cooprider in 1910 in India). Since 1970, however, virtually no new missions have been founded that included medical services. The exception would be some Mennonite Central Committee's short-term assignments. The pattern changed, along with most Protestant denominational policies, due to government-sponsored medical services that characterize the modern nation-state. However, the Seventh-day Adventists, rightly valuing health care as an integral part of the gospel, did not change but continued their practice of integrating medicine and health care more broadly into missions, as Loma Linda University's medical

---

[8]Jacob Ressler's chapter in *Building on the Rock, Various Missionaries* (Scottdale, Penn.: Mennonite Publishing, 1926), pp. 13-17.
[9]Wilbert R. Shenk, *By Faith They Went Out: Mennonite Missions 1850-1999*, Occasional Papers 20 (Elkhart, Ind.: Institute of Mennonite Studies, 2000), p. 87.

training exemplifies. Since 1976, when Mennonite mission agencies and the Mennonite Central Committee formed the Council of International Ministries (CIM), overseas mission and development programs in education and health care are coordinated through CIM.[10]

CONSCIENTIOUS OBJECTION TO WAR AND MENTAL HEALTH

One of the greatest innovations in health care occurred through church initiatives during and following World War II. Conscientious objectors to military service were given the privilege by the U.S. government to work in alternative service to the military, with the drafted men, however, supported by the churches. Many served in mental hospitals. The men saw the dehumanized treatment of the mentally ill—more like animals than human beings.[11] Their two years of service in these state-run institutions left a searing moral impact on their emotions and sense of call to make it better. The story of the great change in mental health care that developed in America over the next decades is largely the story of the Civilian Public Service (CPS) legacy. Church initiatives developed new methods and institutions for care of the mentally ill.

Alex Sareyan tells this moving story in *The Turning Point*.[12] Sareyan lists in appendix C the names of the men who served in Civilian Public Service mental hospitals and who in turn filled out his questionnaire that provided the source for his definitive study. Appendix D lists the mental hospitals in which they served by category: the religious body that had oversight and provided support for the CPS men. Appendix F lists the number of men serving per religious denomination, including the number

---

[10]Ibid., p. 79.

[11]While many features of these institutions were deplorable, they were built originally as mansions with considerable land, and they provided some good features (recreation, farm work and a structured daily schedule) that have been mostly lost in today's hospitalized treatment—or often lack of treatment. See the article by Oliver Sacks, "The Lost Virtues of the Asylum," *New York Review*, September 24, 2009, pp. 50-52.

[12]Alex Sareyan, *The Turning Point: How Persons of Conscience Brought About Major Change in the Care of America's Mentally Ill* (Scottdale, Penn.: Herald Press, 1994), pp. 208-10. A more recent and comprehensive study, with an engaging detailed narrative of the origins of the 1940 Selective Training and Service Act (pp. 9-15) and how the camps were developed and financed (pp. 20-21), is by Steven J. Taylor, *Acts of Conscience: World War II, Mental Institutions, and Religious Objectors* (Syracuse, N.Y.: Syracuse University Press, 2009). This story is told through a PBS film called *The Good War and Those Who Refused to Fight It;* see the website www.pbs.org/itvs/thegoodwar/.

of unaffiliated and unclassified. The total number was 11,996, with Mennonites, Church of the Brethren and Society of Friends constituting 6,969, a significant influence from the historic peace churches. These men and their legacies of testimony and conscientious vision gave rise to a new moral consciousness and vision for the humane treatment of the mentally ill. The minority church was at the forefront of this health care revolution!

The details of this heart-gripping story are too many to recite, but several highlights merit mention.[13] The testimonies and leadership for new forms of mental health treatment resulted in the National Committee for Mental Hygiene that then merged with the Psychiatric Foundation in 1950 to form the National Association of Mental Health (NAMH), which developed goals and protocol for humane treatment. NAMH developed three primary objectives:

- Facilitate the best possible treatment resources for those suffering with mental illness.

- Stimulate research that will lead to the cure and amelioration of mental diseases.

- Promote activities that will lead to the prevention of mental and emotional disorders.

New forms of mental health treatment developed in the following years. Several dozen mental health treatment centers developed under Mennonite leadership in the next several decades,[14] and similar centers (most often initially with day-patient treatment only in the first stages) with hospitals developed later when government funding became available. This impulse, from an ecclesial moral vision for reform of the care of the mentally ill, has had an effect also on other forms of health treatment.

Motivated by justice, shalom and service, numerous health care initiatives emerged over the last century, with Mennonites often at the forefront, especially in integrating services to low-, moderate- and upper-income groups. These services include health care centers, mental health

---

[13]Another important narrative source, especially for the Mennonite Church, which had over a third of the men serving in CPS mental hospitals, is told by Vernon H. Neufeld, ed., *If We Can Love: The Mennonite Mental Health Story* (Newton, Kans.: Faith and Life Press, 1983).

[14]The listing of these, with types of service provided, is narrated by Esther Jost, in *The Mennonite Encyclopedia*, ed. C. J. Dyck and Dennis Martin (Scottdale, Penn.: Herald Press, 1990), 5:578-79.

services, retirement campuses (with low-income housing, assisted living and nursing care), community clinics and disability services.[15]

Disability services among Mennonites began in the 1960s as family members of persons with developmental disabilities pressed church leaders for assistance. Within the context of rural life and love for family, these services developed from Anabaptist values: community, love, service, peace and justice. Administration of these services transitioned through numerous church agencies over the last half-century. In 2011 a Congregational Accessibility Network (CAN) developed as a separate interfaith advocacy organization relating to the National Council of Churches (NCC).[16]

On the larger issue of the U.S. health care system, or better, *industry*, not all health insurance companies are responsive to mental health needs. In an article titled "Health Care and Community" Mark Wenger narrates a story in which a board-certified psychiatrist strongly recommended a church member to be admitted immediately to a local psychiatric center but was denied health insurance coverage by an accountant at the company a thousand miles away. With his pastoral pleading on the phone there was no budge. So they drove forty-five minutes away for E.R. care. Only when the person's employer petitioned (and perhaps threatened) the insurance company was the decision reversed.[17] While progress is underway, the United States has a long way to go to resolve the inequities in health care access, in the priority of mission over margin, and in making shalom and service the motivating factors of entering into and practicing in the health care system. Yet these perspectives and priorities should guide the church as well as the church's witness to the nation, as each seeks to fulfill its moral responsibilities and opportunities.

---

[15]These are coordinated by the Mennonite Health Service Alliance (MHS Alliance), which sponsors various facilities: forty-four retirement centers, eleven developmental disability centers, ten mental health institutions, three general health care facilities and two hospitals. See www.mhsonline.org.

[16]See Paul D. Leichty, "Mennonite Advocacy for Persons with Disabilities," *Journal of Religion, Disability, and Health* 10 (2006): 195-205. In 2010 the Mennonite Medical and Nursing Associations merged to form Mennonite Health Fellowship (MHF), which publishes *Mennonite Health Journal*. Mennonite Health Fellowship, together with the Mennonite Chaplains Association and MHS Alliance, plan an annual health assembly, which with the *Journal* (since spring 2012, online only) serves all these health agencies.

[17]Mark R. Wenger, "Health Care and Community," *Dream Seeker*, autumn 2009, pp. 3-4.

APPENDIX 2

———— ❖ ————

Center for Healing and Hope

ITS MISSION AND CONTRIBUTION

Elkhart County in northern Indiana has a population of about 175,000, with 40,000 uninsured residents. This is not a mere statistic but a call to churches to do something expressive of the church's long history of making health care available to those who need it. In light of these uninsured people's health care needs, if one heeds Jesus' parable of the good Samaritan, churches must act. Congregations must be the friends who let down the paralytic through the roof to Jesus, the healer (Mk 2:1-10). In 1999 the vision and compassion of a nucleus of people thus formed the Center for Healing and Hope (CHH) to meet the urgent care needs—not primary care—of the uninsured, who would otherwise, according to patients polled, go to the E.R. (28 percent), go home and not seek medical care (42 percent), go to a local pharmacy (9 percent) or a range of other responses. Since its founding this center has served thousands, providing for their urgent care health needs (in 2010 alone, 2,791 patients).

The foundational support of this church ministry is threefold, as interdenominational churches work together to make this ministry feasible:

- Ministry partner congregations regularly lift up in prayer the center, its volunteers and the patients.

- Ministry partners encourage their members to participate in the ministry of the center. Ministry teams consist of representatives from supporting congregations of a given clinic. One person on the ministry team serves as a link to CHH. The team has the responsibility to sustain each clinic.

- Ministry partners make a monthly contribution of $50 to $200 to the center, depending on the ability of the partner.

By 2012 the center plans to have five clinics weekly, hosted in three or more different churches.[1] The medical staff and others in supportive roles volunteer their time to make each clinic welcoming, efficient and helpful to those with urgent health care needs. The time period for each clinic's medical services, day or evening, is about three hours. Two medical doctors, a nurse, a greeter and other volunteers in supportive roles are available at each site. Between fifteen and twenty patients may be served in each site. Prescribed drugs are made available at the site, or generic drugs ($4 per month or $10 per quarter or less) may be obtained from a nearby drugstore. Local hospitals have agreed to extend to their doctors serving in this capacity malpractice insurance for any suits. The center has also a policy for those not otherwise covered.

The procedure is as follows: (1) patients arrive, (2) are warmly welcomed by a greeter, and then (3) are shown to a comfortable waiting area; (4) after doing intake, usually by a nurse, (5) the patient is treated by a volunteer doctor. Last, (6) a patient advocate does follow-up, including connecting the patient to a primary care physician or a specialist, if needed. The nurse provides continuity and facilitates record keeping.

Patients are asked to pay a minimal fee of $20, if they are able. If they cannot, ministry partners pick up the fee. If a patient belongs to a supporting congregation and is deemed unable to pay, the patient is given a cMAP card,[2] with which the visit is documented for the congregation's financial remuneration to the clinic. CCH is supported by income from the clinics (patient fees), churches, individual contributions, businesses, grants from foundations, fundraising events and in-kind contributions (donated pharmaceutical and medical supplies, etc.).

More information is available on the website for Center for Healing and Hope (www.chhclinics.org). A similar model of extending medical care to the uninsured is that of Shepherd's Hope in Orlando, Florida.

---

[1] Belmont Mennonite Church is a site for two clinics weekly.
[2] cMAP means Church Medical Assistance Program.

Bibliography

[*Ex Auditu* 21 (2005) has a helpful annotated bibliography on healing, medicine and suffering. Less than one-third of those sources appear in this bibliography, and less than one-third of this bibliography's entries appear in the *Ex Auditu* 21 (2005) bibliography. This book has a wider topical focus and is written six years later. The two bibliographies together provide a rich resource.]

Adler, Jerry, and Jeneen Interlandi. "The Hospital That Could Cure Health Care." *Newsweek*, December 7, 2009, pp. 52-56.

Anderson, Bernhard W. *Out of the Depths*. Philadelphia: Westminster Press, 1983.

Anderson, Ray S. "Healing and the Atonement." Unpublished paper, 1986.

Avalos, Hector. *Health Care and the Rise of Christianity*. Peabody, Mass.: Hendrickson, 1999.

———. *Illness and Health Care in the Ancient Near East: The Role of the Temple in Greece, Mesopotamia, and Israel*. Harvard Semitic Monographs 54. Atlanta: Scholars Press, 1995.

———, Sarah J. Melcher and Jeremy Schipper, eds. *This Abled Body: Rethinking Disabilities in Biblical Studies*. Atlanta: Society of Biblical Literature, 2007.

Bakken, Kenneth L. *The Call to Wholeness: Health as Spiritual Journey*. New York: Crossroad, 1985.

———, and Kathleen H. Hoffeller. *The Journey into God: Healing and Christian Faith*. Minneapolis: Fortress Augsburg, 2000.

———. *The Journey Toward Wholeness: A Christ-Centered Approach to Health and Healing*. New York: Crossroad, 1988.

Barrett, David. "Getting Ready for Mission in the 1990s: What Should We Be Doing to Prepare?" *Missiology: An International Review* 15, no. 1 (January 1987), pp. 3-14.

Barry, Patricia. "The New Face of Health Care: A new system rewards doctors and hospitals for taking better care of patients at lower costs." *AARP Bulletin*, April 1, 2009 (6 print pages). Available at www.aarp.org/health/doctors-hospitals/info-04-2009/the_new_face_of_health_care.html.

Bartel, Dean A., et al. *Supportive Care in the Congregation: Providing a Congregational Network of Care for Persons with Significant Disabilities*. Rev. ed. Harrisonburg, Va.: Mennonite Publishing, 2011.

Barth, Karl. *Church Dogmatics*. Vol. 4, pt. 3.1: *The Doctrine of Reconciliation*. Translated by Geoffrey W. Bromiley. Edinburgh: T & T Clark, 1961.

Bazzana, Giovanni Battista. "Early Christian Missionaries as Physicians: Healing and Its Cultural Value in the Greco-Roman Context." *Novum Testamentum* 51 (2009): 232-51.

Beker, J. Christiaan. *Suffering and Hope: The Biblical Vision and the Human Predicament*. Grand Rapids: Eerdmans, 1994.

Bellah, Robert, et al. *Habits of the Heart: Individualism and Commitment in American Life*. New York: Harper & Row, 1985.

Bennett, Amanda. "The Cost of Hope." *Newsweek*, June 4 & 11, 2012, pp. 52-55.

Bernardin, Joseph Cardinal. *The Gift of Peace: Personal Reflections*. Chicago: Loyola Press, 1997.

Betcher, Sharon V. *Spirit and the Politics of Disablement*. Minneapolis: Fortress, 2007.

Bliss, Edward Jr. *Beyond the Stone Arches: An American Missionary Doctor in China, 1892-1932*. New York: Wiley, 2001.

Boelens, Peter A. "Primary Health Care in an Industrialized Country." In *Transforming Health: Christian Approaches to Healing and Wholeness*. Edited by Eric Ram. Monrovia, Calif.: MARC, 1995.

Boffey, Philip M. Editorial, "Quality Control: The Money Traps in U.S. Health Care." *New York Times*, January 22, 2012, p. SR 12.

Borg, Markus J. *Jesus: A New Vision: Spirit, Culture, and a Life of Discipleship*. San Francisco: Harper & Row, 1987.

Bouma, Hessel, III, et al. *Christian Faith: Health and Medical Practice*. Grand Rapids: Eerdmans, 1989.

Boyd, Gregory A. *Is God to Blame? Beyond Pat Answers to the Problem of Suffering*. Downers Grove, Ill.: InterVarsity Press, 2003.

Bredin, Mark R. *True Beauty: Finding Grace in Disabilities*. Grove Spirituality Series. Cambridge: Grove, 2007.

Brooke, Avery. *Healing in the Landscape of Prayer*. Boston: Cowley, 1996.

Brown, Michael L. *Israel's Divine Healer*. Grand Rapids: Zondervan, 1995.

Brueggemann, Walter. *The Message of the Psalms*. Minneapolis: Augsburg, 1984.

Buller, Cornelius A. "Mutual Aid: Harbinger of the Kingdom?" In *Building Communities of Compassion*. Edited by Willard M. Swartley and Donald B. Kraybill. Scottdale, Penn.: Herald Press, 1998.

Cardenal, Ernesto. *Love*. Translated by Dinah Livingston. New York: Crossroad, 1981.

Carney, Peter M. "Is Greed Good???" Paper presented at a medical ethics conference, University of Notre Dame, Notre Dame, Ind., March 2-4, 2012.

Carter, Erik W. *Including People with Disabilities in Faith Communities: A Guide for Service Providers, Families, and Congregations*. Baltimore, Md./London/Sydney: Paul H. Brookes, 2007.

The Challenge of L'Arche, with introduction and conclusion by Jean Vanier. Minneapolis: Winston Press, 1981.

Chirban, John T. "Healing and Orthodox Spirituality." *Ecumenical Review* 45 (1993): 337-44.

———, ed. *Health and Faith: Medical, Psychological, and Religious Dimensions*. Washington, D.C.: University Press of America, 1991.

Christian Medical Commission. *Healing and Wholeness: The Church's Role in Health*. Geneva, Switzerland: WCC Publications, 1990.

Clapp, Rodney. "Health Money Can't Buy." *Christian Century*, September 22, 2009, p. 45.

Cooper, Elissa. "Why Not College for the Disabled? New Faith-Based School Opens Doors for Young Adults with Intellectual Disabilities." *Christianity Today*, November 2010, pp. 17-19.

Croft, Steven J. L. *The Identity of the Individual in the Psalms*. Sheffield, U.K.: JSOT Press, 1987.

Curtis, Heather D. *Faith in the Great Physician: Suffering and Divine Healing in American Culture: 1860-1900*. Baltimore: Johns Hopkins University, 2007.

Dahood, Mitchell. *Psalms: Introduction, Translation, and Notes*. Anchor Bible. Garden City, N.Y.: Doubleday, 1966.

Dawn, Marva J. *Being Well When We're Ill: Wholeness and Hope in Spite of Infirmity*. Minneapolis: Augsburg, 2008.

Day, Jackson. "The Health Care Debate: Fostering Civil Discussion." *Circuit Rider* 34, no. 3 (2010): 4-6.

Dorien, Gary. "Health Care Fix: The Role of a Public Option." *Christian Century*, July 14, 2009, pp. 12-13.

Downing, Raymond. *Death and Life in America: Biblical Healing and Biomedicine*. Scottdale, Penn.: Herald Press, 2008.

Dueck, Al. "The Church as a Healing Community." *Builder* 41 (1991): 2-8.

Dyck, Sally. "Editorial: Stick to What We Know." *Circuit Rider* 34, no. 3 (2010): 1.

Edwards, Tilden. *Sabbath Time: Understanding and Practice for Contemporary Christians*. New York: Seabury Press, 1982.

Eiesland, Nancy L., and Don E. Saliers, eds. *Human Disability and the Service of God: Reassessing Religious Practices*. Nashville: Abingdon, 1998.

Ervin, Howard M. *Healing: Sign of the Kingdom*. Peabody, Mass.: Hendrickson, 2002.

Ferguson, Everett. *Demonology of the Early Christian World*. New York: Edwin Mellen, 1984.

Ferngren, Gary B. *Medicine and Health in Early Christianity*. Baltimore: Johns Hopkins University Press, 2009.

Fisher, Kathleen M., and Urban C. von Wahlde. "The Miracles of Mark 4:35–5:43: Their Meaning and Function in the Gospel Framework." *Biblical Theological Bulletin* 11 (1981): 13-16.

Flowers, Betty Sue, David Grubin and Elizabeth Meryman-Brunner, eds. *Healing and the Mind: Bill Moyers*. New York: Doubleday, 1995.

Francis, Robert D. "Pursuing the Possible: Religious Voices on Health Care." *Christian Century*, July 14, 2009, pp. 10-12.

Fretheim, Terence E. *The Suffering of God: An Old Testament Perspective*. Philadelphia: Fortress, 1989.

Frost, Evelyn. *Christian Healing*. London: A. R. Mowbray, 1940.

Frykholm, Amy. "Health-Care Option: A Mennonite Plan for Mutual Aid." *Christian Century*, September 22, 2009, pp. 28-31.

Furnish, Victor Paul. *The Love Command in the New Testament*. Rev. ed. Nashville: Abingdon, 2010.

Gager, John. *Kingdom and Community: The Social World of Early Christianity*. Englewood Cliffs, N.J.: Prentice-Hall, 1976.

Gaiser, Frederick J. *Healing in the Bible: Theological Insight for Christian Ministry*. Grand Rapids: Baker, 2010.

———. "'Your Sins Are Forgiven . . . Stand Up and Walk': A Theological Reading of Mark 2:1-12 in the Light of Psalm 103." In Health and Healing. *Ex Auditu: An International Journal of the Theological Interpretation of Scripture* 21. Eugene, Ore.: Wipf & Stock, 2005.

Gawande, Atul. "The Hot Spotters: Can We Lower Medical Cost by Giving the Needed Patients Better Care?" *New Yorker*, January 24, 2011, pp. 41-51.

Gebbie, Kristine M. "Health Care Reform: Get Everyone In!" *Word & World* 30 (2010): 99, 101.

Gellman, Marc. "Bringing the Ancient Word to the Modern World." In *Theological Voices in Medical Ethics*. Edited by Allen Verhey and Stephen E. Lammers. Grand Rapids: Eerdmans, 1993.

Georgi, Dieter. *Remembering the Poor: The History of Paul's Collection for the Poor.* Translated by John Bowden. Nashville: Abingdon, 1992.

Gerstenberger, Erhard S., and Wolfgang Schrage. *Suffering.* Translated by John E. Steely. Nashville: Abingdon, 1980.

Gigliotti, Marcus A. "Qoheleth: Portrait of an Artist in Pain." In *The Bible and Suffering: Social and Political Implications.* Edited by Anthony J. Tambasco. Mahweh, N.J.: Paulist Press, 2002.

Gingerich, James Nelson. "Reflections on Funding Driven and Vision Driven Organizational Health Care Models." Speech at Anabaptist Mennonite Biblical Seminary, Elkhart, Indiana, 2009.

Gingerich, Owen. *God's Universe.* Cambridge, Mass.: Belknap Press of Harvard University Press, 2006.

Ginsburg, Paul B. "Reforming Provider Payment—The Price Side of the Equation." *The New England Journal of Medicine* 365 (2011): 1268-70.

Goldingay, John. *Old Testament Theology: Israel's Life,* vol. 3. Downers Grove, Ill.: IVP Academic, 2009.

González, Justo L. *Faith and Wealth: A History of Early Christian Ideas on the Origin, Significance, and Use of Wealth.* San Francisco: Harper & Row, 1990.

Gowan, Donald E. "Salvation as Healing." In *Ex Auditu* 5 (1989): 1-19.

Granberg-Michaelson, Karin. *Healing Community.* Geneva, Switzerland: WCC Publications, 1991.

Grassi, Joseph A. *Healing the Heart: The Transformational Power of Biblical Heart Imagery.* New York: Paulist Press, 1987.

Green, Joel B. "Healing." In *New Interpreter's Bible Dictionary,* vol. 2. Edited by Katharine Doob Sakenfeld, et al. Nashville: Abingdon Press, 2007, pp. 755-64.

Greenspoon, Leonard. "The Origin of the Idea of the Resurrection." In *Traditions in Transformation: Turning Points in Biblical Faith.* Edited by Baruch Halpern and Jon D. Levenson. Winona Lake, Ind.: Eisenbrauns, 1981, pp. 247-321.

Grundmann, Christoffer H. *Sent to Heal! Emergence and Development of Medical Missions.* Lanham, Md.: University Press of America, 2005.

Haakas, Stanley Samuel. *Health and Medicine in the Eastern Orthodox Tradition.* New York: Macmillan, 1990.

Hall, John Douglas. *God and Human Suffering: An Exercise in the Theology of the Cross.* Minneapolis: Augsburg, 1986.

Hardesty, Nancy A. *Faith Cure: Divine Healing in the Holiness and Pentecostal Movements.* Peabody, Mass.: Hendrickson, 2003.

Hartzler, Rachel Nafziger. *Grief and Sexuality: Life After Losing a Spouse.* Scottdale, Penn.: Herald Press, 2006.

Hauerwas, Stanley. *Hannah's Child: A Theologian's Memoir.* Grand Rapids: Eerdmans, 2010.

———. *Naming the Silences: God, Medicine, and the Problem of Suffering.* Grand Rapids: Eerdmans, 1990.

———. "The Politics of Gentleness: Abled and Disabled." *Christian Century,* December 2, 2008, pp. 28-32.

———, and Jean Vanier. *Living Gently in a Violent World: The Prophetic Witness of Weakness.* Downers Grove, Ill.: InterVarsity Press, 2008.

———, and William H. Willimon. *Resident Aliens.* Nashville: Abingdon, 1989.

Hays, Richard B. *The Moral Vision of the New Testament: Community, Cross, New Creation.* San Francisco: HarperSanFrancisco, 1996.

Heschel, Abraham. *The Prophets.* Evanston and New York: Harper & Row, 1962.

Hilton, Dave. "Global Health and the Limits of Medicine: An Interview with Dave Hilton." *Second Opinion* 18 (1993): 52-68.

Iglehart, John K. "Defining Essential Health Benefits—The View from the IOM Committee." *New England Journal of Medicine* 365 (2011): 1461-63.

Janzen, Waldemar. "Human Wholeness in Biblical Perspective." In *Still in the Image: Essays in Biblical Theology and Anthropology.* Newton, Kans.: Faith and Life Press, 1982.

Johnson, Rick. "Flat-World Health Care." *HealthLeaders* (2009): 28-33.

Jost, Esther. "Mental Health Facilities and Services, North America." In *The Mennonite Encyclopedia.* Edited by C. J. Dyck and Dennis Martin. Vol. 5. Scottdale, Penn.: Herald Press, 1990.

Juhnke, Jim. *Vision, Doctrine, War: Mennonite Identity and Organization in America 1890-1930.* Scottdale, Penn.: Herald Press, 1989.

Jung, Carl. *Answer to Job.* Translated by R. F. C. Hull. Princeton, N.J.: Princeton University Press, 1973.

Kee, Howard Clark. "Medicine and Healing." In *Anchor Bible Dictionary.* Edited by David Noel Freedman et al. Vol. 6. New York: Doubleday, 1992.

———. *Medicine, Miracle, and Magic in New Testament Times.* Cambridge, U.K.: Cambridge University Press, 1986.

Kelley, Henry Ansgar. *The Devil at Baptism: Ritual, Theology and Drama.* Ithaca, N.Y.: Cornell University Press, 1985.

Kelsey, Morton T. *Companions on the Inner Way: The Art of Spiritual Guidance.* New York: Crossroad, 1986.

———. *Healing and Christianity: A Classic Study.* 3rd ed. Minneapolis: Augsburg, 1995.

Kilner, John F., Robert D. Orr and Judith Allen Shelly, eds. *The Changing Face of Health Care: A Christian Appraisal of Managed Care, Resource Allocation, and*

Patient-Caregiver Relationships. Grand Rapids: Eerdmans, 1998.

Klaassen, Walter. "The Anabaptist Tradition." In *Caring and Curing: Health and Medicine in the Western Religious Traditions*. Edited by Ronald L. Numbers and Darrel W. Amundsen. New York: Macmillan, 1986.

Koenig, Harold G. *Medicine, Religion and Health: Where Science and Spirituality Meet*. West Conshohocken, Penn.: Templeton Foundation Press, 2008.

Koontz, Gayle Gerber. "Editorial." *Vision: A Journal for Church and Theology* 8, no. 2 (2007): 3-5.

Kotva, Joseph, Jr., ed. *Healing Health Care: A Study and Action Guide on Health Care Access in the United States*. Anabaptist Center for Health Care Ethics. Scottdale, Penn.: Faith & Life Resources, 2005.

————. "Mutual Aid as 'Practice.'" In *Building Communities of Compassion*. Edited by Willard M. Swartley and Donald B. Kraybill. Scottdale, Penn.: Herald Press, 1998.

Krabill, Willard S., M.D., "The Church and National Health Care Reform." *Mennonite Medical Messenger* 44.3 (July-September, 1993): 7-18.

Kraybill, Donald B., Steven M. Nolt and David L. Weaver-Zercher, *Amish Grace: How Forgiveness Transcended Tragedy*. San Francisco: Jossey-Bass, 2007.

————. *The Amish Way: Patient Faith in a Perilous World*. San Francisco: Jossey-Bass, 2010.

Kreider, Alan. *The Change of Conversion and the Origin of Christendom*. Eugene: Ore.: Wipf & Stock. 2006.

Kushner, Harold S. *When Bad Things Happen to Good People*. New York: Schocken, 1981.

Kydd, Ronald A. N. *Healing Through the Centuries: Models for Understanding*. Peabody, Mass.: Hendrickson, 1998.

Lambrecht, Jan, and Raymond F. Collins, eds. *God and Human Suffering*. Louvain Theological and Pastoral Monographs 3. Grand Rapids: Eerdmans, 1990.

Lammers, Stephen E. "Theology, Medical Ethics, and the Church." In *Theological Voices in Medical Ethics*. Edited by Allen Verhey and Stephen E. Lammers. Grand Rapids: Eerdmans, 1993.

Lapsley, James. *Salvation & Health: The Interlocking Process of Life*. Philadelphia: Westminster, 1972.

Leaman, Tim. "Hard Rock into Springs of Water: Working in Hope." *Mennonite Health Journal* 11, no. 3 (2009): 8-11, 22-26.

Leichty, Paul D. "Mennonite Advocacy for Persons with Disabilities." In *Journal of Religion, Disability, and Health* 10 (2006): 195-205.

Levenson, Jon D. *Resurrection and the Restoration of Israel: The Ultimate Victory of the God of Life*. New Haven, Conn.: Yale University Press, 2006.

Lewis, C. S. *The Problem of Pain.* New York: Macmillan, 1963.

Lind, Millard C. *Yahweh Is a Warrior.* Scottdale, Penn.: Herald Press, 1980.

Luz, Ulrich. "The Significance of the Biblical Witness for Church Peace Action." In *The Meaning of Peace.* Edited by Perry B. Yoder and Willard M. Swartley. Translated by Walter Sawatsky (chap. 20 by Gerhard Reimer). Elkhart, Ind.: IMS, 2001.

Lysaught, M. Therese, and Joseph J. Kotva Jr., eds. *On Moral Medicine: Theological Perspectives in Medical Ethics.* With the assistance of Stephen E. Lammers and Allen Verhey. Grand Rapids: Eerdmans, 2012.

MacNutt, Francis. *Healing.* Notre Dame, Ind.: Ave Maria Press, 1999.

Mahar, Maggie. *Money Driven Medicine: The Real Reason Health Costs So Much.* New York: Harper Collins, 2005.

Martin, Joseph B. *From Alfalfa to Ivy: Memoirs of a Harvard Medical School Dean.* Edmonton, Alberta, Can.: University of Alberta Press, 2011.

Marty, Martin E. Foreword to *Health and Medicine in the Anabaptist Tradition.* Edited by Graydon Snyder. Valley Forge, Penn.: Trinity Press International, 1995.

———, and Kenneth L. Vaux, eds. *Health/Medicine and the Faith Traditions: An Inquiry into Religion and Medicine.* Philadelphia: Fortress, 1982.

Mathews, Susan F. "All for Naught: My Servant Job." In *The Bible and Suffering: Social and Political Implications.* Edited by Anthony J. Tambasco. Mahweh, N.J.: Paulist Press, 2001.

Mbon, Friday. "Deliverance in the Complaint Psalms: Religious Claim or Religious Experience." *Studies in Biblical Theology* 12 (1982): 3-15.

McDermond, J. E. *1, 2, 3 John.* Believers Church Bible Commentary. Scottdale, Penn.: Herald Press, 2011.

McDonough, Mary J. *Can a Health Care Market Be Moral? A Catholic Vision.* Washington, D.C.: Georgetown University Press, 2007.

McGee, John J., and Frank J. Menolascino. *Beyond Gentle Teaching: A Nonaversive Approach to Helping Those in Need.* New York: Plenum Press, 1991.

McGrath, Alister E. *A Life of John Calvin: A Study in the Shaping of Western Culture.* Oxford: Blackwell, 1990.

McKnight, Scot. *A Community Called Atonement.* Nashville: Abingdon, 2007.

McManus, Jim. *The Healing Power of the Sacraments.* Notre Dame, Ind.: Ave Maria, 1984.

Mechanic, Robert E. "Opportunities and Challenges for Episode-Based Payment." *The New England Journal of Medicine* 365 (2011): 777-79.

Meggitt, Justin J. *Paul, Poverty and Survival.* Edinburgh: T & T Clark, 1998.

Meilaender, Gilbert. *Bioethics: A Primer for Christians.* Grand Rapids: Eerdmans, 1996.

Messer, Neil. "Toward a Theological Understanding of Health and Disease." *Journal of the Society of Christian Ethics* 31, no. 1 (2011): 161-78.

Miller, Dean M. "Anointing: An Ancient Rite." *Messenger*, June 1987, pp. 26-27.

Miller, Glen E. *Empowering the Patient: How to Reduce the Cost of Health Care and Improve Its Quality.* Indianapolis: Dog Ear, 2009.

Miller, Kris A. "Streams of Healing: The Theological Frameworks of Prayer for Healing in Three Twentieth-Century Protestant Traditions." Unpublished thesis, Abilene Christian University, 2002.

Moltmann, Jürgen. *The Crucified God: The Cross of Christ as the Foundation and Criticism of Christian Theology.* Translated by R. A. Wilson and John Bowden. New York: Harper & Row, 1974.

———. *The Way of Jesus Christ: Christology in Messianic Dimensions.* Translated by Margaret Kohl. Minneapolis: Fortress, 1993.

Morley, Janet. *All Desires Known.* Wilton, Conn.: Morehouse-Barlow Co., Inc., 1998.

Morris, Charles R. "Health Care for All: Not Easy, Not Cheap, But Possible." *Commonweal*, August 15, 2008, pp. 8-10.

Moyers, Bill. *Healing and the Mind: Bill Moyers.* Edited by Betty Sue Flowers, David Grubin and Elizabeth Meryman-Brunner. New York: Doubleday, 1995.

Muir, S. C. "'Look How They Love One Another': Early Christian and Pagan Care of the Sick and Other Charity." In *Religious Rivalries in the Early Roman Empire and the Rise of Christianity.* Edited by L. E. Vaage. Studies in Christianity and Judaism 18. Waterloo, Ont.: Wilfrid Laurier University Press, 2006.

Mukherjee, Siddhartha. *The Emperor of All Maladies: A Biography of Cancer.* New York: Scribner's, 2010.

Murray, Christopher J. L., and Julio Frenk. "Ranking 37th—Measuring the Performance of the U.S. Health Care System." *The New England Journal of Medicine* 362 (2010): 98.

Murray, Stuart. *Biblical Interpretation in the Anabaptist Tradition.* Scottdale, Penn.: Herald Press, 2000.

Nelson, James Douglas. *Awakening: Restoring Health Through the Spiritual Principles, Shalom, Jesus and the Twelve Step Recovery Program.* Blue Ridge Summit, Penn.: TAB Books, 1989.

Neufeld, Vernon H., ed. *If We Can Love: The Mennonite Mental Health Story.* Newton, Kans.: Faith and Life Press, 1983.

Nickle, Keith F. *The Collection: A Study in Paul's Strategy.* Studies in Biblical Theology 48. London: SCM Press, 1966.

Norberg, Tilda. *Consenting to Grace: An Introduction to Gestalt Pastoral Care.* New York: Penn House Press, 2006.

————, and Robert D. Webber. *Stretch Out Your Hand: Exploring Healing Prayer.* Inver Grove Heights, Minn.: United Church Press, 1990.

Nouwen, Henri J. M. "The Gulf Between East and West." *New Oxford Review,* May 1994.

————. *The Wounded Healer: Ministry in Contemporary Society.* New York: Doubleday, 1972.

Oberlander, Jonathan. "Health Care Policy in an Age of Austerity." *The New England Journal of Medicine* 365 (2011): 1075-77.

Oepke, A. "Ιαομαι." In *Theological Dictionary of the New Testament.* Edited by Gerhard Kittel and Gerhard Friedrich. Vol. 3. Grand Rapids: Eerdmans, 1965, pp. 191-215.

Panikulam, George. *Koinōnia in the New Testament: A Dynamic Expression of Christian Life.* Analecta Biblica 85. Rome: Biblical Institute Press, 1979.

Parsons, Stephen. *The Challenge of Christian Healing.* London: SPCK, 1986.

Patte, Daniel. *Paul's Faith and the Power of the Gospel.* Philadelphia: Fortress, 1983.

Payne, Leanne. *The Healing Presence: Curing the Soul Through Union with Christ.* Grand Rapids: Baker, 1995.

Petsky, Allan S., M.D., Ph.D., Stephen R. Ganthier, B.Sc. and Victor R. Fuchs, Ph.D. "Specialization in Medicine: How Much Is Appropriate?" *The Journal of the American Medical Association,* February 1, 2012, pp. 463-64.

Pfatteicher, Philip H. "Some Early and Later Fathers on the Visitation of the Sick." *Pro Ecclesia* 19, no. 2 (2010): 207-22.

Pilch, John J. "Healing in Mark: A Social Science Analysis." *Biblical Theology Bulletin* 15 (1985): 142-50.

————. *Healing in the New Testament: Insights from Medical and Mediterranean Anthropology.* Minneapolis: Fortress, 2000.

————. "The Health Care System in Matthew: A Social Science Analysis." *Biblical Theology Bulletin* 16 (1986): 102-6.

————. "Understanding Biblical Healing: Selecting the Appropriate Model." *Biblical Theology Bulletin* 18 (1988): 60-66.

Porter, Michael, and Elizabeth Omsted Teisberg. *Redefining Health Care, Creating Value-Based Competition on Results.* Boston: Harvard Business School Press, 2006.

Porterfield, Amanda. *Healing in the History of Christianity.* Oxford: Oxford University Press, 2005.

"Quality, Affordable Health Care for All Americans." In "Patient Protection and Affordable Care Act." September 23, 2011. www.healthcare.gov.

"Reducing Costs, Protecting Consumers: Affordable Care Act on the One Year

Anniversary of the Patient's Bill of Rights," September 23, 2011. www.healthcare.gov.

Reid, T. R. *The Healing of America: A Global Quest for Better, Cheaper, and Fairer Health Care.* New York: Penguin, 2009.

Reno, R. R. "Reforming the Health-Care Reform." *First Things,* June-July 2010, pp. 61-63.

Ressler, Jacob, et al. *Building on the Rock, Various Missionaries.* Scottdale, Penn.: Mennonite Publishing House, 1926.

Reynolds, Thomas E. *Vulnerable Communion: A Theology of Disability and Hospitality.* Grand Rapids: Brazos Press, 2008.

Robertson, Christopher T., Richard Egelhof and Michael Hoke. "Get Sick, Get Out: The Medical Causes of Home Mortgage Foreclosures." *Health Matrix: Journal of Law-Medicine* 18, no. 65 (2008).

Robinson, James M. *The Problem of History in Mark.* Studies in Biblical Theology 21. London: SCM Press, 1957.

Roth, John D. "The Christian and Anabaptist Legacy in Healthcare." In *Healing Healthcare.* Edited by Joseph Kotva Jr. Anabaptist Center for Health Care Ethics. Scottdale, Penn.: Faith & Life Resources, 2005.

Sacks, Oliver. "The Lost Virtues of the Asylum." *New York Review,* September 24, 2009, pp. 50-52.

Saracco, Norberto. "The Holy Spirit and the Church's Mission of Healing." *International Review of Mission* 93, nos. 370, 371 (2004): 413-20.

Sareyan, Alex. *The Turning Point: How Persons of Conscience Brought About Major Change in the Care of America's Mentally Ill.* Scottdale, Penn.: Herald Press, 1994.

Savage, Joseph M. "Shalom and Its Relationship to Health/Healing in the Hebrew Scriptures: A Contextual and Semantic Study of the Books of Psalms and Jeremiah." Ph.D. dissertation, Florida State University, 2001.

Schiefelbein, Kyle K. " 'Receive This Oil as a Sign of Forgiveness and Healing': A Brief History of the Anointing of the Sick and Its Use in Lutheran Worship." *Word & World* 30, no. 1 (2010): 51-62.

Schrage, Wolfgang. "Heil und Heilung im Neuen Testament: Gesammelte Studien." In *Kreuzestheologie und Ethik im Neuen Testament.* Göttingen: Vandenhoeck & Ruprecht, 2004.

Schumpeter. "Getting on the Treadmill." *The Economist,* October 8, 2011, p. 80.

Schwartz, Ted. *Healing in the Name of God: Faith or Fraud?* Grand Rapids: Zondervan, 1993.

Schwartzentruber, Michael. "The Disabled Church." *Gospel Herald,* March 10, 1988, pp. 161-63.

Schweitzer, Albert. *The Quest of the Historical Jesus: A Critical Study of Its Progress from Reimarus to Wrede*. Translated by W. Montgomery. New York: Macmillan, 1906.

Seton, Margaret. "Providing for Those Who Have Too Little." *The New England Journal of Medicine* 365 (2011): 1169-71.

Seybold, Klaus, and Ulrich B. Mueller. *Sickness and Healing*. Translated by Douglas W. Stott. Nashville: Abingdon, 1978.

Shank, David A. "A Prophet of Modern Times: The Thought of William Wade Harris." Unpublished Ph.D. dissertation, Aberdeen, U.K.: Aberdeen University, 1980.

Shenk, Wilbert R. *By Faith They Went Out: Mennonite Missions 1850-1999*. Occasional Papers 20. Elkhart, Ind.: Institute of Mennonite Studies, 2000.

Shillington, George. *2 Corinthians*. Believers Church Bible Commentary. Scottdale, Penn.: Herald Press, 1999.

Shuman, Joel. "Naming Medicine Among the Powers." In Health and Healing. *Ex Auditu: An International Journal of the Theological Interpretation of Scripture* 21. Eugene, Ore.: Wipf & Stock, 2005. "Response" by Stephen Bilynskyj.

Sisson, Jonathan Paige. "Jeremiah and the Jerusalem Conception of Peace." *Journal of Biblical Literature* 105 (1986): 429-42.

Smedes, Lewis B. ed. *Ministry and the Miraculous: A Case Study at Fuller Theological Seminary*. Pasadena: Fuller Theological Center, 1987.

Smith, David H. "A Covenant-Centered Ethic for Medicine." In *Theological Voices in Medical Ethics*. Edited by Allen Verhey and Stephen E. Lammers. Grand Rapids: Eerdmans, 1993.

Snyder, Graydon F. *Health and Medicine in the Anabaptist Tradition*. Valley Forge: Penn.: Trinity Press International, 1995.

Snyder Belousek, Darrin W. *Atonement, Justice, and Peace: The Message of the Cross and the Mission of the Church*. Grand Rapids: Eerdmans, 2012.

Stanger, Frank Bateman. *God's Healing Community*. Wilmore, Ky.: Francis Asbury Society, 1985.

Starfield, Barbara. "America's Healthcare System Is the Third Leading Cause of Death." *Journal of the American Medical Association* 284, no. 4 (2000): 483-85.

Stark, Rodney. "A Double Take on Early Christianity." *Touchstone* 13, no. 1 (2000): 44-47.

———. *The Rise of Christianity: A Sociologist Reconsiders History*. Princeton, N.J.: Princeton University Press, 1996.

Stearns, Richard. *The Hole in Our Gospel*. Nashville: Thomas Nelson, 2010.

Stendahl, Krister. *Paul Among Jews and Gentiles*. Philadelphia: Fortress, 1976.

Swartley, Henry. *Living on the Fault Line: Portrait and Journals of a Church Planter Pastor*. Edited by Willard Swartley. Nappanee, Ind.: Evangel Press, 1992.

Swartley, Willard M. "Biblical Sources of Stewardship." In *The Earth Is the Lord's: Essays on Stewardship*. Edited by Mary Evelyn Jegen and Larry Bruno. New York: Paulist Press, 1978.

———. *Covenant of Peace: The Missing Peace in New Testament Theology and Ethics*. Grand Rapids: Eerdmans, 2006.

———. *Israel's Faith Traditions and the Synoptic Gospels: Story Shaping Story*. Peabody, Mass.: Hendrickson, 1994.

———. *Mark: The Way for All Nations*. Eugene, Ore.: Wipf & Stock, 1999.

———. "Mutual Aid Based in Jesus and Early Christianity." In *Building Communities of Compassion*. Edited by Donald B. Kraybill and Willard M. Swartley. Scottdale, Penn.: Herald Press, 1998.

———. Related articles on Christ's victory over the powers and deliverance ministry in *Even the Demons Submit: Continuing the Ministry of Jesus*. Edited by Loren Johns and James Krabill. Scottdale, Penn.: Herald Press, 2007, pp. 24-40, 108-15, 177, 181-99; *Transforming the Powers: Peace, Justice, and the Domination System*. Edited by Ray Gingerich and Ted Grimsrud. Minneapolis: Fortress, 2006, pp. 96-112, 143-56; *Jesus Matters*. Edited by James Krabill and David W. Shenk. Scottdale, Penn.: Herald Press, 2009, pp. 89-102.

Tada, Joni Eareckson, "Something Greater Than Healing." Interview with Sarah Pulliam Bailey, *Christianity Today*, October 8, 2010, pp. 30-32.

Taylor, Steven J. *Acts of Conscience: World War II, Mental Institutions, and Religious Objectors*. Syracuse, N.Y.: Syracuse University Press, 2009.

Thobaben, James R. *Health-Care Ethics: A Comprehensive Christian Resource*. Downers Grove, Ill.: InterVarsity Press, 2009.

Thomas, John Christopher. "Health and Healing: A Pentecostal Contribution." In Health and Healing. *Ex Auditu: An International Journal of the Theological Interpretation of Scripture* 21. Eugene, Ore.: Wipf & Stock, 2005. "Response" by Rebekah Eklund.

———. "The Spirit, Healing and Mission: An Overview of the Biblical Canon." *International Review of Mission* 93, nos. 370, 371 (2004): 421-42.

Thomas, Leo, with Jan Alkire. *Healing Ministry: A Practical Guide*. Kansas City: Sheed & Ward, 1994.

Thompson, Deanna A. "Suffering Through Lent." *Christian Century*, March 22, 2011, pp. 12-13.

Thurston, Bonnie. *Spiritual Life in the Early Church*. Minneapolis: Fortress, 1993.

Toedtman, James S. "Health Care Reform: 7 Critical Maneuvers." *AARP Bulletin*, December 9, 2009, pp. 12-14.

Toussaint, John. "ThedaCare's Lean Approach to Primary Care." *Medical Home News* 2.6, June 2010, pp. 1, 6-8.

Troxel, Terrie E. "Health Care Reform: Don't Trust It to the Angels!" *Word & World* 30 (2010): 98, 100.

Umble, Jeni Heitt. "Mutual Aid Among the Augsburg Anabaptists." In *Building Communities of Compassion*. Edited by Willard M. Swartley and Donald B. Kraybill. Scottdale, Penn.: Herald Press, 1998.

Vanier, Jean. *Community and Growth*. 2nd ed. Mahwah, N.J.: Paulist Press, 1989.

———. "L'Arche: Its History and Vision." In *The Church and Disabled Persons*. Edited by Griff Hogan. Springfield, Ill.: Templegate, 1983, pp. 52-61.

Verhey, Allen. "Can Medical Ethics Be Christian." In *Theological Voices in Medical Ethics*. Edited by Allen Verhey and Stephen E. Lammers. Grand Rapids: Eerdmans, 1993.

———. "Health and Healing in Memory of Jesus." In Health and Healing. *Ex Auditu: An International Journal of the Theological Interpretation of Scripture* 21. Eugene, Ore.: Wipf & Stock, 2005. "Response" by Dwight Peterson.

———. *Reading the Bible in the Strange World of Sickness*. Grand Rapids: Eerdmans, 2003.

———. *Remembering Jesus: Christian Community, Scripture, and the Moral Life*. Grand Rapids: Eerdmans, 2002. Part 2.

———. "Still Dying Badly." *Christian Century*, November 1, 2011, pp. 22-27.

———, and Stephen E. Lammers, eds. *Theological Voices in Medical Ethics*. Grand Rapids: Eerdmans, 1993.

Vincent, Lori L., Mark L. Vincent, M.D., and Paul J. LeMarbre. *Fighting Disease, Not Death: Finding a Way through Lifelong Struggle*. Indianapolis: Dog Ear, 2011.

Volck, Brian. "Toward a Theology of Disability." *Christian Century*, December 2, 2008, pp. 32-34.

Wallack, Anya Rader. "Single Payer Ahead—Cost Control and the Evolving Vermont Model." *The New England Journal of Medicine* 365, no. 7 (2011): 584-85.

Walls, Andrew F. *The Cross-Cultural Process in Christian History*. Maryknoll, N.Y.: Orbis, 2002.

Walsh, William, and John Langan. "Patristic Social Consciousness: The Church and the Poor." In *The Faith That Does Justice: Examining the Christian Sources for Social Change*. Edited by John C. Haughey. New York: Paulist, 1977.

Waltner, Erland. "Shalom and Wholeness." *Brethren Life and Thought* 29 (1984): 145-51.

Waltner, James H. *Psalms*. Believers Church Bible Commentary. Scottdale, Penn.: Herald Press, 2006.

Weems, Ann. *Psalms of Lament*. Louisville: Westminster/John Knox, 1995.

Weisberg, Jacob. "We Are What We Treat: Fixing Health Care, American Style." *Newsweek*, July 27, 2009, p. 27.

Wenger, Mark R. "Anointing the Sick with Oil in the Mennonite Church: An Exercise in Practical Theology." Ph.D. dissertation, Union Theological Seminary and Presbyterian School of Christian Education, 2000.

———. "Health Care and Community." *Dream Seeker*, autumn 2009, pp. 3-6.

Westermann, Claus. "Peace [Shalom] in the Old Testament." In *The Meaning of Peace*. Edited by Perry B. Yoder and Willard M. Swartley. Elkhart, Ind.: Institute of Mennonite Studies, 2001.

White, Barbara J. "A Nurse's Experience." In *The Changing Face of Health Care*. Edited by John F. Kilner, Robert D. Orr and Judith Allen Shelly. Grand Rapids: Eerdmans, 1998.

Wilkinson, John. *The Bible and Healing: A Medical and Theological Commentary*. Grand Rapids: Eerdmans, 1998.

Williams, Rowan. *Writing in the Dust: Reflections on 11th September and Its Aftermath*. London: Hodder & Stoughton, 2002.

Williams, Tammy. "Is There a Doctor in the House?" In *Practicing Theology: Beliefs and Practices in Christian Life*. Edited by Miroslav Volf and Dorothy C. Bass. Grand Rapids: Eerdmans, 2002.

Wink, Walter. *Engaging the Powers: Discernment and Resistance in a World of Domination*. Minneapolis: Fortress Press, 1992.

Wolfensberger, Wolf. "The Theological Voice of Wolf Wolfensberger." *Journal of Religion, Disability & Health* 4, nos. 2-3 (2001). See especially Wolfensberger's "Response" to the panel of essays, pp. 149-57.

Wolterstorff, Nicholas. *Lament for a Son*. Grand Rapids: Eerdmans, 1987.

Woodman, Josef. *Patients Beyond Borders: Everybody's Guide to Affordable, World-Class Medical Tourism*. Chapel Hill, N.C.: Healthy Travel Media, 2008.

Woolley, Reginald Maxwell. *Exorcism and the Healing of the Sick*. London: SPCK, 1932.

Wright, N. T. *Bringing the Church to the World*. Minneapolis: Bethany House, 1992.

Wuellner, Flora Slosson. *Heart of Healing, Heart of Light: Encountering God Who Shares and Heals Our Pain*. Nashville: Upper Room Books, 1992.

———. *Prayer, Fear, and Our Powers: Finding Our Healing, Release, and Growth in Christ*. Nashville: Upper Room, 1989.

Yoder, John Howard. *Body Politics: Five Practices of the Christian Community Before the Watching World*. Scottdale, Penn.: Herald Press, 1992.

———. *Christian Attitudes to War, Peace, and Revolution*. Grand Rapids: Brazos Press, 2008.

Yoder, Perry B. *Shalom: The Bible's Word for Salvation, Justice and Peace*. Newton, Kans.: Faith and Life Press, 1987.

————, and Willard M. Swartley, eds. *The Meaning of Peace.* 2nd ed. Elkhart, Ind.: Institute of Mennonite Studies, 2001.

Yoder, Sharon. Illustrated by Jolynn Schmucker. *Annie Funk: Lived to Serve, Dared to Sacrifice.* Guy Mills, Penn.: Faith Builders, 2008.

Yong, Amos. *The Bible and Disability: A New Vision of the People of God.* Grand Rapids: Eerdmans, 2011.

Young, Frances. *Face to Face: A Narrative Essay in the Theology of Suffering.* Edinburgh: T & T Clark, 1990.

Zakaria, Fareed. "Africa's New Path." *Newsweek*, July 27, 2009, p. 26.

Zehr, Howard. *Changing Lenses: A New Focus for Crime and Justice.* Scottdale, Penn. and Waterloo, Ont.: Herald Press, 2005.

Zennett, Mary. *Health for US All: The Transformation of U.S. Health Care.* Colorado Springs: Third Day, 2009.

Zoller, Darryl. "The Ministry of Christian Healing." In *Sharing the Practice* 28, no. 1 (winter 2005), pp. 3-5. The theme of this issue is clergy and church health. Other articles are pertinent also.

Websites, cited for topics:

Center for Healing and Hope: www.mchcc.com

Health Care (USA): www.healthcare.gov; www.health-care-reform.net/causedeath.htm; www.circuitrider.com; www.createhealthcarevalue.com; www.createhealth carevalue.com/data/blog/Medical Home News - June 2010.pdf; www.ama-assn .org/ama/pub/about-ama/our-people/member-groups-sections/medical-student -section/advocacy-policy/medical-student-debt.page?; www.aarp.org/health/ doctors-hospitals/info-04-2009/the_new_face_of_health_care.html; www .healthcare.gov/law/full/; www.healthcare.gov/law/resources/reports/patients -bill-of-rights09232011a.html; www.healthcare.gov/law/timeline/index.html; http://bit.ly/insurance-ceos.

Home Mortgage Foreclosures: http://ssrn.com/abstract=1416947

Mennonite Health Services Alliance: www.mhsonline.org

Military Expenditures: www.globalissues.org/article/75/world-militaryspending; http://passionistsinternational.wordpress.com/2011/04/05/global-day-of-action-on-military-spending

Name Index

Scripture Index